Forensic Nursing
2nd Edition

Scope and Standards of Practice

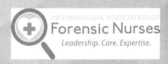

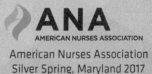

American Nurses Association
Silver Spring, Maryland 2017

American Nurses Association
8515 Georgia Avenue, Suite 400
Silver Spring, MD 20910-3492
1-800-274-4ANA
http://www.Nursingworld.org

International Association of Forensic Nurses
6755 Business Parkway, Suite 303
Elkridge, MD 21075
1-410-626-7805
http://www.ForensicNurses.org/

The American Nurses Association (ANA) is the only full-service professional organization representing the interests of the nation's 3.6 million registered nurses through its constituent member nurses associations and its organizational affiliates. ANA advances the nursing profession by fostering high standards of nursing practice, promoting the rights of nurses in the workplace, projecting a positive and realistic view of nursing, and lobbying the Congress and regulatory agencies on healthcare issues affecting nurses and the public.

The American Nurses Association and International Association of Forensic Nurses (IAFN) are international professional nursing specialty associations. This ANA/IAFN publication, *Forensic Nursing: Scope and Standards of Practice, Second Edition*, reflects the thinking of the forensic nursing specialty on issues that impact forensic nursing practice and should be reviewed in conjunction with state board of nursing policies and practices. State law, rules, and regulations govern the practice of nursing, while *Forensic Nursing: Scope and Standards of Practice, Second Edition*, guides, defines, and directs forensic nurses in the application of their specialization's professional knowledge, skills, and responsibilities.

ISBN-13: 978-1-55810-699-4   SAN: 851-3481   10/2017
eISBNs: 978-1-55810-700-7 (ePDF) ... 978-1-55810-701-4 (EPUB) ...
        978-1-55810-702-1 (Kindle)
First published: October 2017

Contents

Contributors

Forensic Nursing: Scope and Standards of Practice, Second Edition is the product of time, energy, and effort spent reviewing the literature on forensic nursing practice and its governing documents; revising content to reflect current forensic nursing practice; reorganizing content to enhance readability and meet American Nurses Association (ANA) standards; and ongoing collaboration by a highly motivated and dedicated volunteer task force. The Scope and Standards Task Force hosted telephone conferences, used various means of electronic communications to move the document forward, consulted with ANA and International Association of Forensic Nurses (IAFN) staff members, and benefited from the valuable insights of former Scope and Standards of Practice Committee members. Once completed, the draft was reviewed by the IAFN Board of Directors and underwent a public comment period and revision; was submitted to and evaluated by the ANA Committee on Nursing Practice Standards; and lastly, was submitted for approval to the ANA Board of Directors.

Forensic Nursing Scope and Standards Task Force Members

Sara Jennings, DNP, RN, SANE-A, SANE-P, AFN-BC
(Chair, 2016–2017), Virginia

Manager, Bon Secours Forensic Nursing Program (Richmond); two-term Board Member, International Association of Forensic Nurses; President, Virginia Chapter, International Association of Forensic Nurses (2017).

Rachell A. Ekroos, PhD, APRN-BC, AFN-BC
(Chair, 2013–2016), Nevada

Distinguished Fellow, International Association of Forensic Nurses; Evidence Collection Sub-Committee Chair, National Institute of Justice SAFER Act Working Group (2015–2016); Secretary, Patterned Injury Analysis Consensus Body, American Academy of Forensic Sciences Standards Board (2016–2017); Chief Executive Officer, Center for Forensic Nursing Excellence

International; President, Nevada HealthRight; Assistant Professor, School of Nursing, University of Nevada (Las Vegas).

Barbra Bachmeier, JD, MSN, NP-C, Indiana

Advanced Practice Provider/Forensic Nurse Examiner, Emergency Department, Indiana University Health Methodist Hospital (Indianapolis); Chair, Forensic Nursing Committee, Indiana Emergency Nurses Association (2016); Chair, Strangulation Task Force, International Association of Forensic Nurses (2015–2016); Course Director, International Sexual Assault Forensic Examiner Course, Sigma Theta Tau (2016); Board Member, Indiana Coalition Against Domestic Violence (2016–present).

Catherine Carter-Snell, PhD, MN, BScN, RN, SANE-A, ENC-C, Alberta, Canada

Associate Professor of Nursing, Mount Royal University; Co-Founder and Past President, Canadian Forensic Nurses Association; Chapter Co-Author, *Core Curriculum for Forensic Nursing* (IAFN, 2016).

Susan Chasson, JD, MSN, FNP-BC, CNM, SANE-A, Utah

Statewide SANE Coordinator, Utah Coalition Against Sexual Assault; Forensic Nurse, Wasatch Forensic Nurses; President-Elect, International Association of Forensic Nurses (2017).

Kathy Gill-Hopple, PhD, RN, SANE-A, SANE-P, AFN-BC, South Carolina

Forensic Nurse Examiner Coordinator, Medical University of South Carolina; Chair, Tri-County Sexual Assault Response Team (SART).

Georgia Perdue, DNP, FNP-BC, CRNP, Maryland/Delaware

Chapter Co-Author, *Core Curriculum for Forensic Nursing* (IAFN, 2016); Member, Sigma Theta Tau, American Nurses Association, American Association of Nurse Practitioners, Nurse Practitioner's Association of Maryland; Life-Time Member, International Association of Forensic Nurses.

Vikki Vodosia, BSN, RN, SANE-P, Alabama

Nurse Coordinator, CHIPS Center; Member, Alabama Human Trafficking Task Force; Secretary/Treasurer, Alabama Chapter, International Association of Forensic Nurses (IAFN); Abstract Reviewer, IAFN Scientific Assembly (2011–2013); Planner/Organizer, Alabama Chapter, IAFN Annual Conference (2012–2017); Member, IAFN Practice/Poster Abstract Review Team (2016); Member, IAFN Awards Committee (2017); IAFN Nursing Excellence Award (2015–2016).

Kimberly Womack Kasper, DHSc, MSN, ARNP-BC, SANE-A (Board Liaison), New York

Assistant Professor, Graduate Forensic Nursing Program, Duquesne University; President (2015) and Board Member, International Association of Forensic Nurses.

IAFN Staff

Kim Day, RN, SANE-A, SANE-P, South Carolina

Forensic Nursing Director, International Association of Forensic Nurses; Reviewer and Contributor, *Forensic Nursing: Scope and Standards of Practice* (ANA & IAFN, 2017).

Kathleen Maguire, JD, BSN, BS, RN (Task Force Staff Liaison; In-House Editor), Maryland

Certification Director, International Association of Forensic Nurses; Managing Editor, *Journal of Forensic Nursing* (2013–2016); Co-Editor, *Core Curriculum for Forensic Nursing* (IAFN, 2016); Senior Editor, American Nurses Credentialing Center (2006–2013); Former Legal Editor, Bureau of National Affairs; Former Special Consultant, American Bar Association; Senior Legal Researcher, American Association for Justice (1993–present).

Jennifer Pierce-Weeks, RN, SANE-A, SANE-P, New Hampshire

Chief Operations Officer, International Association of Forensic Nurses; Reviewer and Contributor, *Forensic Nursing: Scope and Standards of Practice* (ANA & IAFN, 2017); Past President, International Association of Forensic Nurses; Former Forensic Nursing Program Manager, Colorado Springs, Colorado.

Special Recognition

The members of the Forensic Nursing Scope and Standards Task Force would like to thank Dr. Patricia M. Speck and Dr. Anita Hufft for sharing their invaluable insight and lessons learned during their five-year service on the Committee to Write *Forensic Nursing: Scope and Standards of Practice* (2009).

ANA Staff

Carol J. Bickford, PhD, RN-BC, CPHIMS, FHIMSS, FAAN—Content editor

Joi Morris, BS, CAP-OM—Project coordinator

Lisa M. Myers, Esq.—Legal counsel

Liz Stokes, JD, RN—Ethics consultant

Eric Wurzbacher, BA—Project editor

ANA Committee on Nursing Practice Standards

Danette Culver, MSN, APRN, ACNS-BC, CCRN, Co-Chair

Patricia Bowe, DNP, MS, RN, Co-Chair

Renee Gecsedi, MS, RN

Richard Henker, PhD, RN, CRNA, FAAN

Kirk Koyama, MSN, RN, CNS

Carla Lee, PhD, APRN-BC, CNAA, FAAN, FIBA

Tonette McAndrew, MPA, BSN, RN

Verna Sitzer, PhD, RN, CNS

Tom Blodgett, PhD, MSN, RN-BC, Alternate

Stacy McCall, MSN, RN, IBCLC, Alternate

About the American Nurses Association

The American Nurses Association (ANA) is the only full-service professional organization representing the interests of the nation's 3.6 million registered nurses through its constituent member nurses associations and its organizational affiliates. ANA advances the nursing profession by fostering high standards of nursing practice, promoting the rights of nurses in the workplace, projecting a positive and realistic view of nursing, and lobbying the Congress and regulatory agencies on healthcare issues affecting nurses and the public.

About the International Association of Forensic Nurses

The International Association of Forensic Nurses (IAFN) is a professional organization of nurses who provide specialized health care for patients impacted by violence and trauma. We establish and provide standards of practice and education for forensic nurses. Our members have the knowledge and expertise to decrease the healthcare consequences of violence, improve patient recovery, and lower healthcare costs.

About ANA's Specialty Nursing Standards

Since the late 1990s, ANA has partnered with other nursing organizations to establish a formal process for recognition of specialty areas of nursing practice. This includes the criteria for approving the specialty itself and the scope statement, and an acknowledgment by ANA of the standards of practice for that specialty. Because of the significant changes in the evolving nursing and healthcare environments, ANA's approval of specialty nursing scope statements and its acknowledgment of specialty standards of practice remain valid for five years, starting from the publication date of the documents.

Overview of the Content

Essential Documents of Forensic Nursing

Forensic Nursing: Scope and Standards of Practice, Second Edition, identifies the expectations for the role and practice of the forensic nurse. It builds on the earlier version of this material, published in 2009 by the American Nurses Association (ANA) and the International Association of Forensic Nurses (IAFN). The updated document is meant to define and direct forensic nursing practice in all settings and across all roles. This complex and comprehensive consensus document has been developed with input from the IAFN membership, among others, and uses the ANA framework and guide for scope and standards documents approved by the Congress on Nursing Practice and Economics (ANA, 2010b, 2015b).

The Scope of Forensic Nursing Practice statement (starting on page 1) describes the *who, what, where, when, why*, and *how* of forensic nursing practice. Each of these questions must be answered sufficiently to provide a complete picture of the dynamic and complex practice of forensic nursing and its evolving boundaries and membership. The depth and breadth of an individual forensic nurse's practice—within the total scope of forensic nursing practice—depend upon the nurse's education, experience, role, setting, and the population served.

The Standards of Forensic Nursing Practice, composed of the standards of practice (starting on page 41) and the standards of professional performance (starting on page 57), are authoritative statements of the duties that all forensic nurses—regardless of role, population, or subspecialty—are expected to perform competently. The standards published herein may be used as evidence of the standard of care governing forensic nursing practice, with the understanding that application of the standards is context dependent. The standards are subject to change with the dynamics of the forensic nursing profession and as the specialty and the public develop and accept new patterns of professional practice. In addition, specific conditions and clinical circumstances may affect the application of the standards at a given time (e.g., during a natural disaster or epidemic). The standards are subject to formal, periodic review and revision.

The competencies accompanying each standard are not all-inclusive. The competencies serve as elements that forensic nursing professionals may use to measure professional performance. Whether a particular standard or competency applies depends upon the circumstances. By evaluating their performance, based on these elements, nurses practicing within this particular role, population, and specialty identify opportunities for development and improvement.

Additional Content

To gain an appreciation of the history, content, and context related to *Forensic Nursing: Scope and Standards of Practice, Second Edition*, readers are encouraged to consult the additional content of the previous edition in Appendix B, *Forensic Nursing: Scope and Standards of Practice*.

Audience for this Publication

Forensic nurses in every role and setting comprise the primary audience for this professional resource. Students, interprofessional colleagues, agencies, and organizations will also find this an invaluable reference. In addition, legislators, regulators, legal counsel, and the judiciary will want to examine and reference this content. Finally, the individuals, families, groups, communities, and populations using forensic nursing services can consult this document to better understand what constitutes the specialization of forensic nursing and who forensic nurses are: registered nurses and advanced practice registered nurses.

Licensure and Education of the Registered Nurse

As stated in *Nursing: Scope and Standards of Practice, Third Edition*:

> The registered nurse is licensed and authorized by a state, commonwealth, or territory to practice nursing. Professional licensure of the healthcare professions is established by each jurisdiction to protect the public safety and authorize the practice of the profession. Because of this, the requirements for RN licensure and advanced practice nursing vary widely.

> The registered nurse is educationally prepared for competent practice at the beginning level upon graduation from an accredited school of nursing and qualified by national examination for RN licensure. ANA has consistently affirmed the baccalaureate degree in nursing as the preferred educational preparation for entry into nursing practice.

The registered nurse is educated in the art and science of nursing, with the goal of helping individuals and groups attain, maintain, and restore health whenever possible. Experienced nurses may become proficient in one or more practice areas or roles. These nurses may concentrate on healthcare consumer care in clinical nursing practice specialties. Others influence nursing and support the direct care rendered to healthcare consumers by those professional nurses in clinical practice. Credentialing is one form of acknowledging such specialized knowledge and experience. Credentialing organizations may mandate specific nursing educational requirements, as well as timely demonstrations of knowledge and experience in specialty practice.

Registered nurses may pursue advanced academic studies to prepare for specialization in practice. Educational requirements vary by specialty and educational program. New models for educational preparation are evolving in response to the changing healthcare, education, and regulatory practice environments (ANA, 2015b, p. 41).

Scope of Forensic Nursing Practice

Definition of Forensic Nursing

Forensic nursing is specialized nursing care that focuses on patient populations affected by violence and trauma—across the lifespan and in diverse practice settings. Forensic nursing includes education, prevention, and detection and treatment of the effects of violence in individuals, families, communities, and populations. Through leadership and inter-professional collaboration, the forensic nurse works to foster an under-standing of the health effects, effective interventions, and prevention of violence and trauma in the United States and throughout the world.

Forensic nursing practice is grounded in the rich bio-psycho-social-spiritual education of registered nurses (RNs) and uses the nursing process to assess, diagnose, and treat individuals, families, groups, communities, and popula-tions affected by violence and trauma, and the systems that respond to them. Forensic nursing targets the identification, management, and prevention of intentional and unintentional injuries and death in a global community.

The forensic nurse collaborates with agents in the healthcare, social, and legal systems to investigate and interpret clinical presentations and pathologies by evaluating intentional or unintentional physical and psychological injury and death; describing the scientific relationships between injury and evidence; and interpreting the associated or influencing factors, according to the forensic nursing scope and standards of practice.

The forensic nurse integrates forensic and nursing sciences in the assess-ment and care of populations affected by physical, psychological, or social violence, trauma, or death within the clinical or community environs. Privacy, respect, and dignity characterize the services the forensic nurse provides to those affected by crime, unlawful acts, trauma, and intentional and uninten-tional harm. In addition, the forensic nurse strongly advocates for minimum forensic nursing standards of practice in the care of patients. The International Association of Forensic Nurses (IAFN) in the past provided this definition of forensic nursing: "Forensic nursing is the practice of nursing globally when health and legal systems intersect" (ANA & IAFN, 2009, p. 3).

The following expanded descriptions of both of the scope and the standards of forensic nursing practice reflect the evolution and complexity of this nursing specialty.

Forensic Nursing Scope and Standards of Practice

A specialty organization has a responsibility to its members and to the public it serves to develop the scope and standards of practice for its specialty. The IAFN, the professional organization for forensic nurses, is responsible for developing and maintaining the scope of practice statement and standards that apply to the practice of all forensic nurses. This complex and comprehensive consensus document has been developed with broad input from the IAFN membership, among others, and uses the ANA framework and guide for scope and standards documents (ANA, 2010b, 2015b). *Forensic Nursing: Scope and Standards of Practice, Second Edition*, describes a competent level of forensic nursing practice and professional performance that applies to all forensic nurses.

Description of the Scope of Forensic Nursing Practice

The Scope of Forensic Nursing Practice (starting on page 1) describes the *who, what, where, when, why,* and *how* of forensic nursing practice. Each of these questions must be answered sufficiently to provide a complete picture of the dynamic and complex practice of forensic nursing and its evolving boundaries and membership. The definition of forensic nursing provides a succinct characterization of the "what" of forensic nursing. Forensic nurses are registered nurses (RNs) and advanced practice registered nurses (APRNs) who specialize in forensic nursing to comprise the "who" constituency and have been educated, titled, and maintain active licensure to practice nursing.

Forensic nursing occurs "when" a need exists for forensic nursing knowledge, wisdom, caring, leadership, practice, or education, anytime, anywhere. Forensic nursing occurs in any environment "where" a patient is in need of forensic nursing care, information, or advocacy. The "how" of forensic nursing practice is defined in the ways, means, methods, and manners that forensic nurses use to practice professionally. The "why" is characterized as forensic nursing's response to the changing needs of society to achieve positive patient outcomes in keeping with nursing's social contract with an obligation to society. The depth and breadth of an individual forensic nurse's practice—within the total scope of forensic nursing practice—depends upon the nurse's education, experience, role, setting, and the population being served.

The following definitions are provided for clarity and understanding for our readers:

Patients are persons, clients, families, groups, communities, or populations for whom forensic nurses provide services as sanctioned by state regulatory bodies. This global definition is intended to reflect a proactive focus on health and wellness care rather than a reactive perspective to disease and illness.

Forensic nurses (forensic RNs) are individuals who are academically prepared at the undergraduate or graduate level; licensed by a state, commonwealth, territory, government, or regulatory body to practice as an RN; and have received specialized education and training in forensic nursing.

Advanced practice registered nurses specializing in forensic nursing are APRNs who have received specialized training in forensic nursing and who have:

- Completed an accredited graduate level-education program preparing the nurse for one of the four recognized APRN roles (certified registered nurse anesthetist [CRNA], certified nurse-midwife [CNM], clinical nurse specialist [CNS], or certified nurse practitioner [CNP]);

- Achieved a passing score on a national certification examination that measures APRN-, role-, and population-focused competencies and maintain continued competence as evidenced by recertification in the role and population through the national certification program;

- Acquired advanced clinical knowledge and skills preparing the nurse to provide direct care to patients, as well as a component of indirect care; however, the defining factor for all APRNs is that a significant component of the education and practice focuses on direct care of individuals;

- Grounded their practices in the competencies of RNs by demonstrating a greater depth and breadth of knowledge, a greater synthesis of data, increased complexity of skills and interventions, and greater role autonomy;

- Obtained educational preparation to assume responsibility and accountability for health promotion and/or maintenance as well as the assessment, diagnosis, and management of patient problems, which includes the use and prescription of pharmacologic and non-pharmacologic interventions;

- Demonstrated clinical experience of sufficient depth and breadth to reflect the intended license; and

- Obtained a license to practice as an APRN in one of the four APRN roles: CRNA, CNM, CNS, or CNP (APRN Joint Dialogue Group, 2008).

The forensic nurse, regardless of licensure or setting, provides expert, holistic, patient-centered, and trauma-informed care. Patients who have experienced trauma are at risk for both short- and long-term health sequelae, and are vulnerable to re-traumatization when receiving care that does not routinely take into account the effect of trauma on health. With training and expertise in providing care through a trauma-informed lens, the forensic nurse understands the criticality of establishing an unbiased, developmentally appropriate rapport with the patient. Trauma-informed rapport-building involves creating an environment of nurse–patient trust and support; addressing cultural, historical, and gender issues; and giving the patient a voice in their care. The forensic nurse is keenly aware of potential safety issues—before, during, and after the patient's medical–forensic examination and discharge—and plans accordingly in collaboration with professionals from other disciplines.

The forensic nurse's scope of practice ranges from providing care for the patient's bio-psycho-social needs, to maintaining patient privacy and confidentiality, to collecting and documenting evidence, to testifying in a legal proceeding. To perform this specialized practice, the forensic nurse works with an interdisciplinary team composed of medical professionals, community and systems-based advocates, social services workers, faith community leaders, law enforcement personnel, and legal practitioners.

The forensic nurse's goal is to provide quality nursing care to the forensic patient from the initial point of contact to proffering testimony in a courtroom setting, when necessary. The forensic nurse contributes to positive patient outcomes, improved law enforcement investigations, and just legal proceedings. To capture a sense of the specialized work that is forensic nursing, the IAFN collaborated with documentary filmmakers to present a series of vivid vignettes involving forensic nurses practicing in diverse settings. (See Appendix A: Resources, IAFN & Seedworks Films, 2011, 2012.)

Development and Function of the Standards of Forensic Nursing Practice

The Scope of Forensic Nursing Practice Statement is accompanied by the Standards of Forensic Nursing Practice, which consist of the Standards of Practice and the Standards of Professional Performance. These are authoritative statements of the duties that all forensic nurses—regardless of role, population, or subspecialty—are expected to perform competently. The standards published herein may serve as evidence of the standard of care, with the understanding that application of the standards depends upon context. The standards are subject to change with the dynamics of the nursing profession and the forensic nursing specialty as new patterns of professional practice are developed and accepted by the forensic nursing community and the public at-large. In addition, specific conditions and clinical circumstances may affect the application of standards at a given time (e.g., during a disaster or epidemic). As with the scope of practice statement, the standards are subject to formal, periodic review and revision.

Standards of Practice for Forensic Nurses

The Standards of Practice for Forensic Nurses describe a competent level of forensic nursing care as demonstrated by the critical-thinking model known as the nursing process. The nursing process includes the components of assessment, diagnosis, outcomes identification, planning, implementation, and evaluation. Accordingly, the nursing process encompasses significant actions taken by registered nurses and forms the foundation of the nurse's decision-making.

Standard 1. Assessment

The forensic nurse collects pertinent data and information relative to the patient's health, death, or the situation.

Standard 2. Diagnosis

The forensic nurse analyzes the assessment data to determine actual or potential diagnoses, problems, and issues.

Standard 3. Outcomes Identification

The forensic nurse identifies expected outcomes for a plan individualized to the patient or the situation.

Standard 4. Planning

The forensic nurse develops a plan that prescribes strategies to attain expected, measurable outcomes.

Standard 5. Implementation

The forensic nurse implements the identified plan.

Standard 5A. Coordination of Care

The forensic nurse coordinates care delivery.

Standard 5B. Health Teaching and Health Promotion

The forensic nurse employs strategies to promote health and a safe environment.

Standard 6. Evaluation

The forensic nurse evaluates progress toward attainment of goals and outcomes.

Standards of Professional Performance for Forensic Nurses

The Standards of Forensic Nursing Professional Performance describe a competent level of behavior in the professional role, including activities related to ethics, culturally congruent practice, communication, collaboration, leadership, education, evidence-based practice and research, quality of practice, professional practice evaluation, resource utilization, and environmental health. All forensic nurses are expected to engage in professional role activities, including leadership, that is appropriate to their education and position. For their professional actions, forensic nurses are accountable to themselves, their patients, their peers, and ultimately, society.

Standard 7. Ethics

The forensic nurse practices ethically.

Standard 8. Culturally Congruent Practice

The forensic nurse practices in a manner that is congruent with cultural diversity and inclusion principles.

Standard 9. Communication

The forensic nurse communicates effectively in all areas of practice.

Standard 10. Collaboration

The forensic nurse collaborates with patient, family, and other key stakeholders in the conduct of nursing practice.

Standard 11. Leadership

The forensic nurse leads within the professional practice setting and the profession.

Standard 12. Education

The forensic nurse seeks knowledge and competence that reflects current nursing practice and promotes futuristic thinking.

Standard 13. Evidence-Based Practice and Research

The forensic nurse integrates evidence and research findings into practice.

Standard 14. Quality of Practice

The forensic nurse contributes to quality nursing practice.

Standard 15. Professional Practice Evaluation

The forensic nurse evaluates one's own and others' nursing practice.

Standard 16. Resource Utilization

The forensic nurse utilizes appropriate resources to plan, provide, and sustain evidence-based nursing services that are safe, effective, and fiscally responsible.

Standard 17. Environmental Health

The forensic nurse practices in an environmentally safe and healthy manner.

The Function of Competencies in Standards

The competencies that accompany each standard may be evidence of compliance with the corresponding standard. The list of competencies is not exhaustive. Whether a particular standard or competency applies depends upon the circumstances. For example, a nurse providing care for a patient who is unconscious and critically ill and who, unaccompanied by family members, arrived at the hospital by ambulance has a duty to collect comprehensive data pertinent to the patient's health (Standard 1. Assessment). However, under the attendant circumstances, that nurse may not be expected to "[a]ssess[ ] family dynamics and impact on the patient's health and wellness" (one of Standard 1's competencies). In the same instance, Standard 5B. Health Teaching and Health Promotion might not apply at all.

Evolution of Forensic Nursing

The milestones in the development of forensic nursing practice that are listed on the following/next page underscore the importance of this nursing practice specialty in identifying, managing, and preventing intentional and unintentional injuries in a global community. In addition, forensic nursing practice has traditionally provided a role in assessing and providing care for victims, suspects, the accused, and perpetrators of crime, trauma, and intentional harm, particularly those who have a mental or emotional disorder related to the commission of a crime or unlawful act.

Milestones of Forensic Nursing Practice

These key events highlight the critical steps in the development and formalization of forensic nursing:

1948	Article V in the Universal Declaration of Human Rights declares: "No one shall be subjected to torture or to cruel, inhuman or degrading treatment or punishment" (United Nations, 1948).
1975	John Butt, MD, chief medical examiner in Alberta, Canada, recognizes the registered nurse as a valuable resource to the field of death investigation (Lynch & Duval, 2011).
1984	The U.S. Surgeon General identifies violence as a public health issue and healthcare providers as key agents in ameliorating the effects of violence in our communities (Koop, 1986).
1990	Virginia Lynch, RN, Forensic Clinical Nurse Specialist, conceptualizes and operationalizes the role of the forensic nurse examiner (Lynch, 1990).
1991	The ANA publishes a position paper, asserting that violence against women is a nursing practice issue (ANA, 1991).
1991	The American Academy of Forensic Sciences recognizes forensic nursing as a scientific discipline (Lynch & Duval, 2011).

1992	The IAFN is established as the first professional nursing organization for forensic nurses (IAFN, 2017a).
1995	ANA's Congress of Nursing Practice recognizes forensic nursing as a specialty practice area (ANA & IAFN, 1997).
1997	ANA and IAFN jointly publish the first edition of the *Scope and Standards of Forensic Nursing Practice* (ANA & IAFN, 1997).
2001	IAFN develops and publishes *Sexual Assault Nurse Examiner (SANE) Education Guidelines* (IAFN, 2015).
2004	IAFN develops and publishes *Core Competencies for Advanced Practice Forensic Nursing* (IAFN, 2004).
2005	IAFN publishes the first issue of *Journal of Forensic Nursing*.
2009	ANA and IAFN jointly publish the first edition of *Forensic Nursing: Scope and Standards of Practice* (ANA & IAFN, 2009).
2009	IAFN develops and publishes *Forensic Nurse Death Investigator (FNDI) Education Guidelines* (IAFN, 2013a).
2012	IAFN develops and publishes the *Intimate Partner Violence Nurse Examiner Education Guidelines* (IAFN, 2013b).
2015	IAFN publishes the *Core Curriculum for Forensic Nursing* (Price & Maguire, 2015).
2017	ANA and IAFN jointly publish *Forensic Nursing: Scope and Standards of Practice, 2nd Edition.*

Forensic nurses continue to create and disseminate new and existing evidence-based and research-informed knowledge, encourage collaboration among nurses and specialty practices, and promote interprofessional collaboration. The IAFN, the professional organization for forensic nurses, serves an integral role in the continued development of forensic nursing practice across settings, roles, and populations. The IAFN supports the forensic nurse

- In the development of international professional networks;
- Through the recognition and expansion of the unique aspects of forensic nursing practice;
- Through the provision of innovative, evidence-based forensic nursing education;
- In the establishment of the scope and standards of forensic nursing practice;

- In the creation of credentialing processes for forensic nurses; and
- In the development of the core curriculum for forensic nursing.

Forensic nursing is a multifaceted and complex specialty practice. Its responsibilities, functions, roles, and skills derive from general nursing practice, yet the specialty of forensic nursing has developed in accordance with its distinctive practice environments and populations. Forensic nursing practice, concerned primarily with individuals and populations affected by violence and trauma, their families, communities, and the systems that respond to them, may include but is not limited to

- Assessment, diagnosis, identification of outcomes, planning, implementation, evaluation of, and scientific inquiry about human, programmatic, and system responses to injury and interventions following injury to individuals, families, groups, communities, cultures, and environments;
- Identification of the pathology of intentional or unintentional injury in persons who are living or deceased;
- Episodic care for populations affected by trauma, including those legally defined as victims, suspects, the accused, and perpetrators;
- Recognition, collection, packaging, preservation, and transfer of specimens/samples holding potential evidentiary value within the legal system;
- Participation in the generation, dissemination, and use of evidence-based research in forensic nursing practice delivered to patients, communities, and systems;
- Utilization of formative and summative evaluation processes in forensic nursing roles and environments internationally;
- Administration, organization, and coordination of the forensic nursing role in programs, systems, and environments where forensic nurses practice;
- Involvement and influence in both internal and external systems where professional and societal regulation of forensic nursing practice affect public health and safety;
- Development and support of local, regional, and global public policy to support public health as it relates to injury or death and the prevention of injury in a variety of cultures and communities;
- Promotion of and accountability to the ethical principles and vision of ethical practice within forensic nursing;

- Development and implementation of professional and community education programs of interest to forensic nurses that address prevention and interventions in primary, secondary, and tertiary settings; and

- Development and promotion of interprofessional collaboration between the forensic nurse and other professionals—such as community and systems-based advocates, forensic scientists, and legal professionals—in all roles and practice environments.

Prevalence of Forensic Nurses

The National Sample Survey of Registered Nurses (NSSRN), which the Health Resources and Services Administration (HRSA) of the U.S. Department of Health and Human Services (DHHS) conducts approximately every four years, does not report the number of nurses who work within the forensic nursing specialty (DHHS, HRSA, 2010). The survey focuses on educational background, primary/secondary employment setting, primary/secondary position, job satisfaction, salaries, and additional demographic characteristics.

Because forensic nurses serve populations affected by trauma or violence—which are not limited to one setting and are not represented by a specific patient demographic—forensic nurses remain one of the most diverse groups of clinicians in the nursing profession (e.g., patient populations served, practice settings, and forensic healthcare services provided). This unique dynamic confounds the ability of a survey such as the NSSRN to capture accurate practice data specific to forensic nursing. In addition, as the NSSRN reveals, many RNs hold both a part-time and a full-time position (>12%) or multiple part-time positions (another 14%), further confounding the difficulty of identifying unique specialty practices (DHHS, HRSA, 2010). Although more than 3,700 members currently comprise the IAFN (2017a), this number cannot be extrapolated as representative of the total number of nurses who work full-time, part-time, or intermittently as forensic nurses.

Populations Served by Forensic Nurses

Forensic nurses care for and treat individuals, families, groups, communities, and populations in systems where intentional and unintentional injuries occur. These include but are not limited to patients who have been

- Victims, suspects, the accused, or perpetrators of interpersonal violence (e.g., child abuse, elder and vulnerable person abuse, intimate partner abuse and assault, sexual abuse/assault, gang violence, human trafficking);

- Victims, suspects, the accused, or perpetrators of incidents involving human factors (e.g., occupational accidents, motor vehicle collisions, acts of terrorism, forensic-related deaths) (Harris, 2013); and

- Victims of natural causes of trauma and population evacuation (e.g., seismic or weather-related disasters).

Forensic nurses address the forensic healthcare needs of some of society's most vulnerable, marginalized, and often disadvantaged populations, both living and deceased (e.g., children; individuals with congenital and developmental disabilities; LGBTQI—or "Two Spirit" individuals; residents of institutions; patients with mental illness; and individuals who are substance users, homeless, trafficked, or incarcerated). Forensic nurses also respond to community forensic healthcare needs by concentrating on programmatic and systems change (e.g., in the event of threats to public health and safety, responding to environmental hazards with death and mass-casualty incident investigations, providing forensic nursing programs and education, and participating in policy and program development and legislation).

Forensic nurses possess both fundamental and specialized nursing knowledge and skills, including an understanding of the healthcare, social, and legal systems, and knowledge about forensic and public health sciences. Forensic nurses collaborate with professionals in health, social, governmental, and legal systems to investigate and interpret clinical presentations and pathologies. Forensic nurses accomplish this by evaluating physical and psychological injury, whether intentional or unintentional, describing the scientific relationships of the injury and potential evidentiary items, and interpreting the factors that influence them.

Settings for Forensic Nursing Practice

Forensic nurses provide care throughout the domains of nursing practice, administration, education, research, and consultation (ANA & IAFN, 1997, 2009; IAFN, 2004). Furthermore, forensic nurses practice independently and collaboratively as needed in various settings whenever and wherever health and legal issues intersect. Forensic nurses also interact with other systems in healthcare, community, and legal environments, including the following:

- Hospital and pre-hospital settings and clinics

- Long-term care, skilled nursing, and rehabilitation settings

- Legal or investigative arenas

- Commercial, not-for-profit, and non-profit organizations

- Governmental organizations and programs
- Educational and industrial settings
- Residential and correctional institutions

The systems where forensic nurses practice vary, depending on location, funding sources, community standards, and legal influences, and include but are not limited to the following:

- Tribal health-First Nations, native, indigenous populations
- Health care (e.g., hospitals, surgery centers, community clinics)
- Investigative (e.g., medical examiner, coroner, law enforcement agencies, regulatory agencies)
- Judicial (e.g., criminal, civil, and family courts)
- Correctional (e.g., jails, prisons, and detention centers)
- Public sector (e.g., military, local, state, provincial, and federal agencies)
- Social services (e.g., child/adult protective services, advocacy centers)
- Educational (e.g., K–12 schools, colleges, universities)
- Private sector (e.g., industries, agencies, firms)
- International organizations (e.g., World Health Organization [WHO])

In addition, forensic nurse entrepreneurs establish businesses reflecting their forensic nursing practice and consultation expertise. Forensic nurses also serve on local, regional, national, and international advisory boards and working groups to establish best practices, build consensus, and enact change to better serve and represent populations affected by violence and trauma.

The *core* of forensic nursing specifies the definitions, roles, behaviors, and processes inherent in forensic nursing practice. The *boundaries* of forensic nursing are both internal and external with sufficient resilience to adapt to changing societal needs and demands. The *intersections* reflect where the boundaries of forensic nursing practice overlap with those of other professional groups by virtue of nursing's unique application of a common body of knowledge, environment, and focus. *Specialization* in forensic nursing incorporates a multitude of subspecialty areas specific to the forensic health needs of patients in communities and across settings, populations, and systems.

Regardless of the practice setting, the forensic nurse integrates knowledge of nursing science, criminal justice, public health, the forensic sciences, and the phenomena related to violence and trauma across the life span in providing forensic health care to patients, families, communities, and populations.

Roles and Practices of the Forensic Nurse

Forensic nursing roles and practices vary across settings, populations served (e.g., pediatric, adult, older adult), and the type of violence or trauma experienced (e.g., sexual abuse, intimate partner violence [IPV], violence resulting in death). Thus, forensic nursing practices may be described based on setting, population, type of violence, or a combination thereof, in addition to the specific role of the nurse (e.g., clinician, researcher, educator, medicolegal death investigator). For example, forensic nursing roles may include clinical practice, education, administration, research, and consultation in any one or more of the following focal areas of violence or injury:

- Sexual violence

- Intimate partner violence (IPV)

- Physical abuse, maltreatment, and neglect

- Interpersonal violence

- Elder and vulnerable person abuse

- Violence resulting in death

- Intentional and unintentional injury or death

- Mass disaster

- Violence as a global healthcare issue affecting individuals, families, groups, communities, and systems

Forensic nursing specifically responds to the specialized needs of populations affected by violence and trauma as seen in the following four examples.

Forensic Nursing and Sexual Assault

One well-known domain in forensic nursing practice is responding to the trauma of sexual assault and abuse and intervening through actions in systems to mitigate the impact of sexual violence on individuals, families, groups, communities, and society. In a variety of settings—including emergency departments, clinics, and coroner/medical examiner offices—forensic nurses provide care for patients who have experienced sexual assault.

In 2015, the IAFN published updated guidelines for the education of the nurse practicing in the role of sexual assault nurse examiner (SANE) (IAFN, 2015). The forensic nurse who has completed this specialized education is an expert in history-taking, assessment, identification of injury, treatment of trauma response and injury, documentation (written and photographic) and collection of samples for forensic analysis and its management, emotional and social support required during a post-trauma evaluation and examination, and the documentation of injury and the testimony required to bring such cases through the legal system (IAFN, 2015; Speck & Peters, 1999).

As outlined in the 2015 *Sexual Assault Nurse Examiner (SANE) Education Guidelines*, another distinct aspect of the SANE role is the use of a patient-centered and legally objective approach, integrating patient advocacy and observation; recognition of specific injury related to sexual assault; sample collection for forensic analysis; mitigation of and protection against adverse health outcomes, including vicarious trauma; and identification of community resources to support the patient reporting sexual assault (IAFN, 2015). Accordingly, a forensic nurse practicing in the role of a SANE has education reflecting specialized knowledge about legal systems, forensic evidence, ethics, pathophysiology, injury and potential for injury, reproductive health, epidemiology, technology, psychology associated with sexual assault, along with targeted training about the unique patient population served.

The SANE is responsible for representing the patient encounter to the courts and society. This may include the evaluation and treatment of the forensic patient's health status and bio-psycho-social-spiritual responses; the health and forensic assessment, including history taking, identification of injury, specimen collection, and evidentiary outcomes; as well as the systems response in the courts and the community-at-large to the sexual assault.

Forensic Nursing and Intimate Partner Violence (IPV)

Forensic nurses are also providing care and working with patients who are victims of IPV. Intimate partner violence encompasses the continuum of violent and abusive experiences in which multiple variations of harm, neglect, abuse, and violence occur between people in intimate relationships (IAFN, 2013b). IPV is a serious health issue, and the Institute of Medicine (IOM) has called for professional healthcare organizations to develop guidelines that will better inform clinicians about violence and abuse (IOM, 2002). The U.S. Department of Health and Human Services (DHHS) has since provided guidelines for Women's Preventative Services that include screening and counseling for domestic violence, and the Patient Protection and Affordable Care Act of 2010 (Pub. L. No. 111-148, 111–148, 124 Stat. 119) includes provisions for routine screening and counseling of domestic or interpersonal violence.

In 2013, IAFN published *Intimate Partner Violence Education Guidelines* to inform the education needs for forensic nurses working with patients who have experienced IPV. As described in *Intimate Partner Violence Education Guidelines* (IAFN, 2013b), the forensic nurse's role in providing the medical–forensic evaluation of the patient requires application of the nursing process (assessment, diagnosis, outcomes identification, planning, implementation, and evaluation) to the care delivered. The forensic nurse who provides care to patients who are victims of IPV employs a holistic and comprehensive approach (IAFNb, 2013). This approach integrates addressing IPV from a trauma-informed model of care (Harris & Fallot, 2001), including documentation and photography; recognition of specific injuries related to IPV; mitigation of and protection against adverse health outcomes, including vicarious trauma; and identification of community resources to support the patient (IAFN, 2013). The forensic nurse also provides education to healthcare professionals, collaborative partners, and the public on the dynamics and effects of IPV (IAFN, 2013b).

Forensic Nursing and Medicolegal Death Investigation

Forensic nurses involved in medical death investigation bring nursing skills of observation, data collection, and analysis to the determination of manner and cause of death. One objective of the forensic nurse in this setting is to advocate for the forensic patient (the deceased) through the application of nursing skills and knowledge. Forensic nurses have an obligation to consider health promotion beyond the present investigation, using the outcomes of death. The forensic nurse investigating death promotes health among colleagues, families, and communities of the deceased through the manner and tone of investigation. The forensic nursing role includes the preservation of dignity, caring, and protection of human rights even after death.

The forensic nurse death investigator (FNDI) meets the unique forensic needs of individuals served by the medical examiner/coroner system and other regulatory agencies investigating deaths. These nurses have additional education and clinical preparation in conducting a death investigation and forensic evaluation. The FNDI strives to ensure that a competent forensic evaluation and death scene investigation are conducted in all situations. To achieve this goal, the FNDI applies nursing knowledge and the nursing process in all aspects of death investigation, including assessment of the scene, medical–forensic evaluation of injuries, collection/evaluation of specimens, and care of survivors.

In 2013, IAFN published guidelines for the education of the FNDI (IAFN, 2013b). As described in the *Forensic Nurse Death Investigator Education Guidelines* (IAFN, 2013a), the nursing process (assessment, diagnosis, outcomes identification, planning, implementation, and evaluation) applies to forensic investigation in three separate stages:

1. Investigation of the death;

2. Investigation of the decedent's family and/or survivors; and

3. Effects on the community (Wooten, 2003).

These components are interrelated and dynamic, much like the human DNA strand. The six steps of the nursing process are interwoven in the different elements of the FNDI role. They include actions such as assessing the scene at a death, planning for additional sample collection, implementing referrals when caring for survivors, and evaluating all actions taken during an investigation (IAFN, 2013a). The FNDI also uses the nursing process to assess the needs of the community and implement a plan to support and educate community members as needed (Vessier-Batchen, 2007).

Forensic Nursing and Psychiatric–Mental Health/Correctional Settings

Forensic nursing includes the psychiatric–mental health nurse who applies knowledge of psychiatric principles and nursing theory to the care of persons in acute care, community-based, or correctional settings who have psychological or mental disorders (Shives, 2011). The psychiatric nurse may encounter patients who, by virtue of their emotional or mental disorder, commit or are likely to commit crimes or trauma against themselves or others.

The forensic nurse in a psychiatric–mental health setting possesses particularized knowledge and competencies in the assessment, care, and evaluation of individuals with mental disorders as they relate to criminal behavior. The forensic nurse applies principles of forensic psychiatry and nursing to clinically assess, evaluate, and treat individuals or populations with crime-related mental disorders. In addition, the forensic nurse possesses expertise in providing care for patients with mental disorders in secure settings and refining that care to minimize the patient's risk of victimization, self-injury, or injury to others (Mason & Mercer, 1996).

Diversity of Forensic Nursing Skills

Forensic nurses provide direct services to individuals, families, groups, communities, and populations; they affect the systems where they function. In addition, forensic nurses provide consultative services to nursing, medical, social, and other healthcare and legal professionals and entities. Moreover, forensic nurses provide factual and expert court testimony regarding both intentional and unintentional injury of the living or the deceased.

The forensic nurse develops and evaluates programs of care related to intentional and unintentional injury, crime, victimization, violence, abuse, death, and exploitation at the individual, community, state, provincial, district, regional, national, and international levels. For example, the RN practicing in a risk management department in a hospital setting develops protocols for the collection of data and responses to indicators of patient or staff risk in the healthcare setting, including injuries, preventable deaths, and other issues related to safety. In contrast, the forensic nurse working in a healthcare setting uses forensic nursing expertise (e.g., knowledge of medical and scientific investigation, sample collection/preservation, and intentional and unintentional injury) in the clinical investigation of injury and trauma and liability of crime-related trauma affecting specific populations, such as older adults, persons with disabilities (Humphreys & Campbell, 2011), or those who die unexpectedly.

Although the forensic nurse and the risk management nurse collaborate across legal, social, and healthcare systems to provide evidence-based data that support solutions to risk, the forensic nurse has particular expertise in cases relevant to a legal action, such as, but not limited to, homicide, sexual assault, intimate partner violence, or child maltreatment. Unlike the risk management nurse, the forensic nurse has specialized knowledge to identify indicators of criminal activity and risk for injury and is educated to distinguish intentional from unintentional trauma or injury. Although a risk management nurse would focus on the epidemiological trail of a virus or bacterium in an open system, the forensic nurse would focus on the evidence of intentional harm by individuals or groups that contribute to the spread of infection or epidemic (e.g., biohazardous contamination, HIV/AIDS).

The nurses in these two roles may work in collaboration or the forensic nurse may be the designated investigator in the healthcare system when intentional harm is suspected. The forensic nurse may also serve in a consultative, administrative, or leadership role for the institution when intentional harm is suspected (e.g., unexpected or clustered death). The forensic nurse is able to recommend measures to mitigate the opportunity for intentional harm in systems that are willing to implement changes to reduce risk.

Individual forensic nursing practice clearly differs according to both the nurse's experience and educational preparation, and the characteristics of the patient population. Other major factors include the cultural, social, and legal systems in the forensic nursing practice setting.

The following list conveys examples of the significant diversity of skills of the forensic nurse:

- Application of public health and forensic principles to the RN's practice, including bio-psycho-social-spiritual aspects of forensic nursing care in the scientific investigation/evaluation, diagnosis, treatment, and prevention of trauma and/or death of victims, suspects, the accused, and perpetrators, including the measurement of outcomes and outputs of the practice;

- Development and implementation of systems relevant to forensic nursing, including the development of systems that care for individuals, families, groups, and communities in relation to injury, both intentional and unintentional; the care of individuals, families, groups, communities, or populations involved with criminal and civil justice systems; and the measurement of the quality and safety of outcomes;

- Development of quality forensic nursing care strategies through evidence-based practice and inquiry to determine injury causation and identify measures to prevent injury and death, both intentional and unintentional;

- Development, analysis, and implementation of health policy relevant to forensic nurses and patient populations in forensic settings;

- Development and implementation of ethically sound, evidence-based, and culturally relevant processes within forensic nursing settings and systems;

- Development, analysis, reporting, and dissemination of relevant forensic data, evidence-based outcomes, and outputs;

- Identification, collection, and organization of data relevant to forensic nurses;

- Provision of testimony, both fact and expert, in judicial settings, competency hearings, civil and family hearings, and other venues;

- Design, evaluation, reporting, implementation, and dissemination of evidence-based and peer-reviewed research relevant to forensic nurses;

- Analysis of outcomes and influence in justice systems and on legislation that pertains to forensic nursing practice and healthcare quality, safety, outcomes, and outputs;

- Consultation with nursing practice communities and the interprofessional communities of medicine, legal systems, advocacy agencies, governments, and their agents;

- Interprofessional collaboration with justice, political, and social systems, and the individuals who work within those systems;

- Interprofessional education regarding forensic nursing practice;

- Leadership, administration, and management within forensic and healthcare settings;

- Medical–forensic histories for the purpose of diagnosis, treatment, and/or referral;

- Evaluation of crime scenes and trauma within settings relevant to the forensic nurse;

- Analysis of forensic health care through continuous quality review processes;

- Provision of ethical, safe, evidence-based, direct patient care related to injury, crime, victimization, violence, abuse, and exploitation;

- Provision of safe, evidence-based forensic mental health care;

- Collection and preservation of samples and items with potential legal/evidentiary value;

- Integration of evidence-based and evidence-informed forensic nursing practice to improve the care of patients globally; and

- Creation and implementation of forensic nursing systems and environments to improve the quality of forensic patient care, safety, and outcomes.

Ethics and Forensic Nursing Practice
Forensic Nursing Applications of the Code of Ethics for Nurses

The current edition of *Code of Ethics for Nurses with Interpretive Statements* ("the Code") (ANA, 2015a) serves as the ethical framework in nursing regardless of practice setting or role, and provides guidance for nurses now and into the future. The nine provisions of the Code explicate the key ethical concepts and actions for all nurses in all settings in the following context:

> *Code of Ethics for Nurses with Interpretive Statements* (the Code) establishes the ethical standard for the profession and provides a guide for nurses to use in ethical analysis and decision-making. . . . The Code arises from the long, distinguished, and enduring moral tradition of modern nursing in the United States. It is foundational to nursing theory, practice, and praxis in its expression of the values, virtues, and obligations that shape, guide, and inform nursing as a profession (ANA, 2015a, p. vii).

The Code also describes the ethical characteristics of the professional nurse:

> Individuals who become nurses, as well as the professional organizations that represent them, are expected not only to adhere to the values, moral norms, and ideals of the profession but also to embrace

them as a part of what it means to be a nurse. The ethical tradition of nursing is self-reflective, enduring, and distinctive. A code of ethics for the nursing profession makes explicit the primary obligations, values, and ideals of the profession. In fact, it informs every aspect of the nurse's life (ANA, 2015a, p. vii).

Detailed descriptive interpretive statements for each of the nine provisions of the Code are available at http://www.nursingworld.org/codeofethics. The following examples demonstrate how the ethical provisions of the Code (ANA, 2015a, p. v) can be applied to forensic nursing:

Provision 1. **The nurse practices with compassion and respect for the inherent dignity, worth, and unique attributes of every person.**

Karen is working with a statewide sexual violence council to develop a new medical–forensic examination documentation form. The current form only allows for documenting "male" or "female." She requests that the revised form include not only dichotomous sexual identity options but also additional options so patients who so identify may feel both acknowledged and accepted when disclosing a sexual assault.

Provision 2. **The nurse's primary commitment is to the patient, whether an individual, family, group, community, or population.**

While obtaining the initial history from a patient who reports having been sexually assaulted, Anna assesses the patient as being at high risk for HIV exposure. Anna recognizes that HIV prophylaxis is time-sensitive. To ensure her care is patient centered, she alters the order of the forensic-medical–forensic examination to provide the patient with HIV prophylaxis, delaying the collection of samples for forensic analysis until after the patient receives HIV prophylactic medications.

Provision 3. **The nurse promotes, advocates for, and protects the rights, health, and safety of the patient.**

Peter is providing care to a patient who discloses being strangled during a fight with her boyfriend. Peter identifies strangulation as one of several significant risk factors for lethal intimate partner violence (IPV). Additionally, he understands the dynamics of IPV and the associated health consequences. He discusses with the patient the risks to her health and safety in her present relationship, safety plans with her for when she is discharged, and educates her about services available in the community, including safe housing at a local domestic violence shelter.

Provision 4. The nurse has authority, accountability, and responsibility for nursing practice; makes decisions; and takes action consistent with the obligation to promote health and to provide optimal care.

Megan provides training to all local law enforcement agencies on the frequency of strangulation in intimate partner violence incidents, how to ask victims whether strangulation has occurred, the health consequences, and the need for proper medical evaluation, documentation, and treatment in the event of strangulation.

Provision 5. The nurse owes the same duties to self as to others, including the responsibility to promote health and safety, preserve wholeness of character and integrity, maintain competence, and continue personal and professional growth.

Pamela completed the initial medical–forensic evaluation on a two-year-old boy who was severely beaten by his father one week ago. She had been checking on the child in the pediatric intensive care unit every day. The child was pronounced brain dead, taken off life support, and died today. Pamela has a son the same age. She has been experiencing nightmares and has been irritable with her colleagues. Pamela realizes she is experiencing signs of vicarious trauma. She consults her supervisor and requests to be taken off call until she can see a therapist, life coach, or other employee assistance person.

Provision 6. The nurse, through individual and collective effort, establishes, maintains, and improves the ethical environment of the work setting and conditions of employment that are conducive to safe, quality health care.

Sam leads a monthly journal club for his forensic nursing unit. The forensic nurses review a journal article and discuss how they might use the information to enhance the unit's response to violence and trauma, improve patient care, or inform testimony in court cases.

Provision 7. The nurse, in all roles and settings, advances the profession through research and scholarly inquiry, professional standards development, and the generation of both nursing and health policy.

Maria has been studying how nurse death investigators affect the family grief process. She has submitted her findings for publication.

Provision 8. The nurse collaborates with other health professionals and the public to protect human rights, promote health diplomacy, and reduce health disparities.

Kim, who works for a hospital's SANE program, is an active member of the Latino community. Although Latinos comprise 30% of the town's population, only 5% of the patients who report sexual assault are Latino. Kim creates focus groups in her community to identify why Latinos are not reporting. She also provides staff education to enhance cultural knowledge and skills and improve care and services to Latino patients.

Provision 9. The profession of nursing, collectively through its professional organizations, must articulate nursing values, maintain the integrity of the profession, and integrate principles of social justice into nursing and health policy.

The International Association of Forensic Nurses worked to support the passage of the Violence Against Women Act 2013, which for the first time, provides in-statute protections against discrimination based on sexual orientation or gender identity.

Ethical Principles and Priorities of Forensic Nurses

Despite the diversity of patient populations served, practice settings, and forensic and healthcare services provided, all forensic nurses share skills and a body of knowledge related to the identification, assessment, and analysis of forensic patient data. Forensic nurses apply a unique combination of processes rooted in nursing science, the forensic sciences, and public health to care for patients, families, communities, and populations. Because human worth is the philosophical foundation upon which forensic nursing is based, the practice of forensic nursing is consistent with *Code of Ethics for Nurses with Interpretative Statements* (ANA, 2015a), *Vision of Ethical Practice* (IAFN, 2008), and *ICN Code of Ethics for Nurses* (International Council of Nurses [ICN], 2012).

Accordingly, forensic nurses demonstrate an awareness of, and an adherence to, regional and international laws governing their practice. Forensic nurses uphold ethical principles promoted by the nursing profession that protect the rights of, and advocate for, individuals, families, groups, and communities in the systems that respond to these patients. The forensic nurse seeks evidence-based and evidence-informed resources related to the health, safety, legal, and ethical issues involving the forensic patient. Forensic nurses deliver services in a non-judgmental and non-discriminatory manner that is sensitive to the diverse cultural needs of the patient and the community.

The forensic nurse practices with compassion and respect for the uniqueness of patients, including the moral and legal rights associated with self-determination within forensic settings and systems. Forensic nurses collaborate to address the forensic health needs of the patient. When conflicting situations arise (e.g., from bias, prior victimization, addiction, vicarious trauma, or interprofessional situations), forensic nurses examine the conflicts between personal and professional values, strive to preserve the patient's best interest, and preserve their professional integrity by establishing and respecting boundaries.

Nurses have a lifelong commitment to learning and maintaining professional competence. This includes self-evaluation, coupled with peer review, to ensure the nurse's forensic nursing practice meets the highest standard. Forensic nurses are required to have knowledge of matters that are relevant to the current forensic nursing scope and standards of practice, including topical issues related to forensic nursing and nursing ethics (i.e., professional, clinical, and organizational ethics), including concerns and controversies.

Forensic nurses participate in the advancement of practice through administration, education, and knowledge development—as well as development of healthcare policy and professional standards—and dissemination of knowledge germane to forensic nursing practice. This may come from shared domains in nursing (such as public health, genetics, and genomics) or other professions (such as medicine, clinical forensic medicine, public health, and the forensic sciences).

Most importantly, the forensic nurse has responsibilities to the public to respond appropriately to improve access to forensic nursing care and bring social change that creates a world without violence (ANA, 1991, 2010a, 2015a; CNA, 2008b; IAFN, 2008; ICN, 2012).

Levels of Forensic Nursing Practice
RNs Specializing in Forensic Nursing

The forensic nurse is a registered nurse (RN) who is licensed and authorized by a state, commonwealth, or territory to practice nursing. Each jurisdiction establishes professional licensure of the healthcare professions to protect the public safety and authorize the practice of that profession. Because of this, the requirements for RN and APRN licensure vary widely. The RN is educationally prepared for competent practice at the entry level upon graduation from an accredited diploma, associate, baccalaureate, or master's degree nursing program and is qualified by national examination (e.g., National Council Licensure Examination for Registered Nurses, known as NCLEX-RN) for RN licensure. The licensing jurisdiction then grants the legal title of registered nurse, shortened to RN, allowing nurses to use the RN credential after their name as long as their license remains in an active status. The ANA has consistently affirmed the baccalaureate degree in nursing as the preferred educational preparation for entry into nursing practice in the United States.

The RN is educated in the art and science of nursing with the goal of helping individuals, families, groups, communities, and populations attain, maintain, and restore health whenever possible. Experienced nurses may become proficient in one or more practice areas or roles and may elect to concentrate on care of the patient in clinical nursing practice specialties (e.g., forensic nursing). Others influence nursing and support the direct clinical care rendered to patients. Credentialing is one form of acknowledging such specialized knowledge and experience (e.g., SANE-A®, SANE-P®). Credentialing organizations (e.g., Commission for Forensic Nursing Certification) may mandate specific nursing educational requirements as well as timely demonstrations of knowledge and experience in the specialty practice.

RNs seeking to practice forensic nursing may pursue advanced academic studies to prepare for specialization in forensic nursing. Educational requirements vary by subspecialty (e.g., sexual assault, intimate partner violence, death investigation), employer requirements, and academic educational program. New models for forensic nursing educational preparation are evolving in response to the changing healthcare, education, and regulatory practice environments.

A continued commitment to the forensic nursing profession requires forensic nurses to remain involved in continuous learning, thereby strengthening individual practice within varied settings (see Standard 12. Education, page 64). Participation in civic activities, membership in and support of professional associations, collective bargaining, and workplace advocacy also demonstrate forensic nursing commitment. Forensic nurses commit to their profession by using their skills, knowledge, and abilities to act as visionaries; promoting safe practice environments; and supporting resourceful, accessible, and cost-effective delivery of health care to serve the ever-changing needs of the population.

The forensic nurse develops, promotes, and implements evidence-based practice for individuals, families, groups, communities, and populations within systems. In addition, the forensic nurse engages in research and formative and summative program evaluation in systems of care for victims, suspects, the accused, and perpetrators, and the complex health problems associated with violence, criminal acts, and associated trauma for individuals, families, groups, and communities. Health promotion activities provided by the forensic nurse emphasize the identification and prevention of violence and the resulting trauma and injury—as well as the systems changes necessary to respond to this complex patient phenomenon in all types of communities.

Forensic nurses who pursue advanced education at the graduate or doctoral level may select programs and courses of study that do not prepare them for licensure and recognition as an APRN. As may the RN who specializes in forensic nursing, the graduate level-prepared forensic nurse who specializes in forensic nursing may also seek credentialing as a form of acknowledging specific knowledge and experience (e.g., AFN-BC). Credentialing organizations, such as the American Nurses Credentialing Center (ANCC), may mandate specific nursing and forensic nursing educational requirements as well as timely demonstrations of knowledge and experience in the specialty practice.

Advanced Practice Registered Nurses Specializing in Forensic Nursing

Another evolution of nursing practice was the development of educational programs to prepare nurses for advanced practice in direct care roles. These advanced practice registered nurse (APRN) roles include certified registered nurse anesthetists (CRNAs), certified nurse midwives (CNMs), clinical nurse specialists (CNSs), and certified nurse practitioners (CNPs). Each has a unique history and context, but all share a focus on direct care to individual patients. Advanced Practice Registered Nurse is a regulatory title and includes the four roles listed above. State law and regulation further define criteria for licensure for the designated APRN roles. The need to ensure patient safety and access to APRNs by aligning education, accreditation, licensure, and certification is shown in the Consensus Model for APRN Regulation: Licensure, Accreditation, Certification, and Education (APRN JDG, 2008).

APRNs specializing in forensic nursing hold master's or doctoral degrees, have attained expanded and specialized knowledge and skills specific to forensic nursing practice, and are licensed, certified, and approved to practice in their roles as a CNS, nurse practitioner, nurse anesthetist, or CNM. The APRN must obtain a minimum of a graduate degree in nursing with an emphasis in an acknowledged specialty area (e.g., family nurse practitioner) for the prevention of trauma and the diagnosis and treatment of illnesses and responses to trauma, violence, and injury or death.

The APRN specializing in forensic nursing collaborates with criminal/civil justice and healthcare professionals to care for, diagnose, treat, and provide follow-up care for patients affected by injury or death. The APRN diagnoses, treats, and manages acute illness and chronic responses to injury or death in individuals, groups, and communities in the context of the medicolegal system. The APRN prescribes medications and develops healthcare interventions within the scope of practice defined by professional organizations, regulatory agencies (e.g., state board of nursing), and institutions. The health promotion activities of the APRN specializing in forensic nursing emphasize the identification and prevention of risks associated with violence, trauma, and injury or death in systems that respond to the care of patients. An APRN who specializes in forensic nursing and gains advanced forensic education may also apply for and achieve Advanced Forensic Nursing Board Certification (AFN-BC) through the ANCC.

Educational Preparation for Forensic Nursing

Historically, registered nurses have refined and developed their forensic nursing skills through clinical practice and continuing education. Today, five primary routes exist for preparation in forensic nursing (Burgess, Berger, & Boersma, 2004):

1. *Continuing education coursework*—Nurses gain additional skills and knowledge about topics of interest to forensic nurses through continuing education courses.

2. *Certificate programs*—These provide content that is relevant to the forensic nurse, establish entrance requirements and often include clinical internships that result in a certificate detailing the completion of coursework.

3. *Undergraduate nursing education*—Undergraduate academic programs in accredited schools of nursing offer electives, minors, or concentrations in forensic nursing that contribute to a degree in nursing.

4. *Graduate nursing education*—Formal graduate study enhances the knowledge and skills acquired in baccalaureate and prelicensure nursing programs. Following matriculation and completion of the forensic core content and prescribed forensic clinical experiences, the forensic nurse receives a master's or doctoral degree in nursing with a specialization in forensic nursing science.

5. *Post-doctoral education or fellowships*—Formal forensic nursing core content and prescribed forensic clinical experiences enhance the specific content and skills acquired in the terminal nursing degree programs. The programs may award diplomas.

Universities, schools of nursing, community colleges, and continuing education providers offer formal educational opportunities for the specialty of forensic nursing at all academic levels. Entry-level schools of nursing offer introductory classes as electives. Accredited academic institutions offer degrees and certificates at graduate levels. Some forensic nursing education is provided by local, state, provincial, or federal governmental agencies, as well as by entrepreneurs. The IAFN (2004) has published core domains, content, and performance measures in an outline of the curriculum for nurse educators and forensic nurses in practice. Entry-level forensic nursing practice requires completion of a basic nursing program leading to licensure as a RN coupled with specialized forensic nursing education (e.g., elective courses, continuing education, and certificate and certification programs).

The principles of forensic nursing education are rooted in nursing science, public health, and forensic sciences (Speck, 2000). Forensic nursing education focuses on conditions and outcomes that are specific to forensic patients who are involved or potentially involved with the legal system as either victims, the accused, suspects, or perpetrators. Specialized components of education include the following:

- Unique forensic terminology;
- Intentional and unintentional injury;
- Prevention;
- Identification, diagnosis, treatment, and management of patients who include individuals, families, groups, communities, and systems;
- Psychology and psychopathology;
- Victimology;
- Sample collection and preservation;
- Photo documentation; and
- The scientific investigation of death.

The forensic nurse brings all the expertise of the professional nurse to the practice of forensic nursing. Forensic nursing practice is summarized in the concepts of Wounding and Healing, Ethics, and Evidence, coupled with a fundamental understanding of the law and legal processes (WHEEL); these principles are essential to the comprehensive practice of forensic nursing (Speck, 2000).

To remain current in clinical practice and knowledgeable about advancements in technology and legal issues that bear on the practice of forensic nursing, a forensic nurse has a lifelong commitment to learning. Several states or provincial governments mandate continuing education for the forensic nurse to maintain licensure and certification. Education that is current and reflects evidence-based and evidence-informed practice is necessary to ensure safe healthcare delivery and advocacy for forensic patients and employers. Annual conferences, professional meetings held for forensic nursing interest groups, and educational programs and scientific publications serve as educational resources for practitioners at all levels of education and document the practitioner's experience in the forensic nursing specialty. Issues such as differences in judicial processes among local, state, provincial, regional, national, and international venues; dissemination of advances in the forensic sciences and forensic nursing science; and the evolutionary revisions to healthcare standards pose educational challenges to the forensic nurse of the future.

Specialty Certification in Forensic Nursing

Forensic nurses demonstrate competence to the public through education and recognition of their pursuit of excellence in practice. Certification in forensic nursing is a priority for the specialty. Certification demonstrates practice competencies and skills that reflect evidence-based practice. The forensic nurse exhibits expertise in a forensic nursing role through a credentialing process designed to recognize nursing experience in the clinical arena coupled with additional education and validation of knowledge. The forensic nurse acquires and maintains formal credentials available through certifying bodies in the forensic nursing specialty. The forensic nurse contributes to the evidence-based and research-informed knowledge, practice standards, and establishment of criteria for specialty certification.

Certification offers tangible recognition of professional achievement in a defined functional or clinical area of nursing, such as advanced forensic nursing (e.g., AFN-BC), sexual assault nursing (e.g., SANE-A® or SANE-P®), or medicolegal death investigation (e.g., D-ABMDI, F-ABMDI). Through these credentialing processes, forensic nurses earn credentials recognized by the profession and the public at-large. These processes include board certification by examination or by portfolio. The portfolio process for credentialing includes education, clinical hours of practice, peer evaluation of clinical competency, and demonstration of theoretical knowledge.

Professional Competence in Forensic Nursing Practice

"The public has a right to expect [forensic] RNs to demonstrate professional competence throughout their careers" (ANA, 2015b, p. 213). The forensic nurse is individually responsible and accountable for maintaining professional competence. "Regulatory agencies define minimal standards of competence to protect the public. The employer is responsible and accountable to provide a practice environment that is conducive to competent practice. Assurance of competence is the shared responsibility of the profession, individual nurses, professional organizations, credentialing and certification entities, regulatory agencies, employers, and other key stakeholders (ANA, 2014)" (ANA, 2015b, p. 213). The forensic nursing specialty nursing organization also is responsible to shape and guide the processes for ensuring the competence of the forensic nurse.

Evaluating Competence

Competence in forensic nursing practice can be evaluated by the individual nurse (self-assessment), nurse peers, and nurses in the roles of supervisor, coach, mentor, or preceptor. In addition, other aspects of forensic nursing performance may be evaluated by professional colleagues and patients.

Evaluation of competence involves the use of tools to capture objective and subjective data about the individual's knowledge base and actual performance. Those tools must be appropriate for the specific situation and the desired outcome of the competence evaluation. "However, no single evaluation tool or method can guarantee competence" (ANA, 2014, p. 6).

"Ongoing discussions and research on the definitions, meaning, evaluation, and relationship of competence and competency in educational and organizational literature inform nursing professionals about these topics (Hodges, 2010; Levine & Johnson, 2014)" (ANA, 2015b, p. 25). IAFN joins ANA in supporting this important work in the definition, measurement, and validation of nursing and healthcare professional competencies and values major contributions as work associated with the following:

- Evidence-based nursing (Melnyk, Gallagher-Ford, Long, & Fineout-Overholt, 2014);

- Interprofessional competencies (Interprofessional Education Collaborative Expert Panel [IECEP], 2011);

- Leadership competencies (ANA Leadership Institute, 2013); and

- Cultural competence (Guidelines for Implementing Culturally Competent Nursing Care) (ANA, 2015b, p. 45; Douglas et al., 2014) and competencies (ANA, 2015b, pp. 69–70).

Leadership in Forensic Nursing

The ANA recognizes nurse leaders as nurses who "do more than delegate, dictate, and direct" (ANA, 2016). Forensic nurse leaders operate within all nursing practice levels and settings and help advance forensic nursing philosophies and science in patient care, nursing, public health, the forensic sciences, and healthcare policy as it relates to the patient health outcomes.

As researchers, educators, forensic nurse leaders further the understanding of how violence affects the lives of individuals, families, groups, and communities. Forensic nurse leaders conduct research in forensic nursing practice, programs, and processes in global settings for the purposes of recognizing patterns of injury in patient populations, developing new care methodologies, and disseminating the evidence base to guide forensic nursing practice. As administrators, forensic nurse leaders create new, patient-centered models of care for victims of violence while meeting the legal needs of the criminal justice system. Finally, forensic nurse leaders are active at local, state, provincial, national, and international levels of government to advocate for both the needs of their patients and for policies that recognize that violence is a preventable healthcare problem.

International Context of Forensic Nursing

During the past decade, health care and the profession of nursing have undergone dramatic changes worldwide. Various nursing organizations have developed ethical codes to guide all nurses in their nursing practice setting (ANA, 2015a; CNA, 2008b; IAFN, 2008; ICN, 2012). Evolving professional and societal needs and expectations necessitate further clarity regarding the scope of practice for the nurse. Similarly, the demand for the credentialing of nurses in specialty practice mandates consistent and standardized processes for defining the focus and competencies of specialty practice (American Board of Nursing Specialties, 2016; ANA, 2010b, 2015b).

ANA has responded with updated versions of the three documents that provide the foundation of nursing practice in the United States: the *Code of Ethics for Nurses with Interpretive Statements* (2015a), *Nursing: Scope and Standards of Practice, Third Edition* (2015b), and *Nursing's Social Policy Statement: The Essence of the Profession* (2010a). The Canadian Nurses Association (CNA) affirmed similar changes with its adoption of the *Joint Position Statement: Scopes of Practice* (Canadian Medical Association, CNA, & Canadian Pharmacists Association, 2003) and *Advanced Nursing Practice: A National Framework* (CNA, 2008a).

These and other documents, such as the CNA's *Framework for the Practice of Registered Nurses in Canada* (2015), Australia's National Nursing and Nursing Education Taskforce's *National Specialisation Framework for Nursing and Midwifery* (2006), and the ICN's *Position Statement: Scope of Nursing Practice* (2013), delineate the boundaries of professional nursing practice and provide a framework within which nursing specialties globally can establish role expectations across all settings, including practice, education, administration, and research. The organization and content of these documents—as well as the expansion and evolution of the forensic nursing specialty internationally (Schober & Affara, 2006)—have necessarily altered the format and content of the scope and standards of forensic nursing practice.

Forensic Nursing: Scope and Standards of Practice, Second Edition, defines and comprehensively describes forensic nursing as a specialty and provides direction for continued progress and recognition internationally. Designated as a nursing specialty in 1995 by the ANA, forensic nursing represents the response of nurses to the swiftly changing healthcare environment and to the global challenges of caring for victims, suspects, the accused, and perpetrators of intentional and unintentional injury. The scope of forensic nursing practice exists within flexible boundaries across diverse settings and populations. Forensic nurses care for individuals, families, groups, and communities whose status or care is, in part, determined by legal or forensic issues. These patients present in a variety of settings, including in healthcare, educational, legal, legislative, and scientific systems.

The practice of all professional nurses now includes many of the concepts previously deemed unique to the forensic nursing specialty, including violence, prevention of injury and death, victimization, abuse, and exploitation. As the body of knowledge and the skill sets identified as unique to forensic nursing expand, so does the practice of forensic nursing. The statement of the specialty's scope and standards of practice is intended to serve as a foundation for legislation and regulation of forensic nursing and for the development of institutional policies and procedures in settings in which forensic nurses practice. Given rapid changes in healthcare trends and technologies, the standards in this document are intended to be dynamic, nimble, and visionary, allowing flexibility in response to emerging issues and practices of forensic nursing both nationally and internationally.

Professional Trends and Issues in Forensic Nursing
Forensic Nursing Education

Patients' forensic healthcare needs and the care environment are increasingly complex. Nurses and forensic nursing specialists must make critical decisions, be adept at using a variety of sophisticated medical and forensic technology and information management systems, coordinate care among a variety of professional and community agencies, lead change from within their organizations, and affect national policy. Consequently, nursing students need to develop a broader range of competencies in the areas of health policy and healthcare financing (including understanding health insurance and reimbursement for forensic healthcare services), community and public health, leadership, quality improvement, and information management and systems thinking, in addition to becoming excellent clinicians (IOM, 2011).

According to the IOM (2011), to meet this demand, nurses should achieve higher levels of education, while educational systems and other stakeholders should support seamless academic progression and endorse innovative ways for nursing students to achieve their degrees through online, virtual, simulated, and competency-based learning. Curricula design should adequately prepare entry-level nurses and center on optimal patient outcomes. Schools of nursing must also build their capacities to prepare more graduate level-prepared students to assume roles in advanced practice, leadership, teaching, and research (IOM, 2011).

Nursing as a profession continues to face dilemmas in entry into practice, recognition of the autonomy of APRNs, maintenance of competence, complexity of multistate licensure, and the appropriate educational credentials for licensure and professional certification. Forensic nurses have a professional responsibility to maintain competence in their area of practice. Employers who provide opportunities for professional development and continuing education promote a positive practice environment in which nurses can maintain and enhance their skills and competencies.

This is an exciting time of progress and evolution for interprofessional education. According to the American Association of Colleges of Nursing (AACN), interdisciplinary education is "[a]n educational approach in which two or more disciplines collaborate in the learning process with the goal of fostering interprofessional interactions that enhance the practice of each discipline" (1995, p. 1). Students from differing professions learn what each brings to the healthcare team and how each needs to foster communication, collaboration, conflict resolution, and mutual respect before graduation and entry into practice.

Forensic nursing educational programs continue to grow as an increasing number of accredited universities and colleges worldwide develop master's and doctoral curricula in the specialty of forensic nursing (AACN, 2006, 2008). Master's and doctoral education programs reflect the expanding scientific evidence base of forensic nursing. Forensic nursing education follows the trends for specialties using distance learning based on advanced technology, electronically supported simulations, and telemedicine. This trend supports access to education for and by forensic nursing graduate students in remote locations worldwide and improves access to quality forensic nursing care to the patient populations residing in remote communities. Future forensic nurses will assume leadership positions and create new venues for forensic nursing practice, such as entrepreneurial endeavors and legislative representation. Future forensic nurses will widely influence nursing practice and policy; elements of forensic nursing content will continue to be woven throughout nursing coursework at all levels of nursing education.

Technological Advances

Technology can drive effectiveness and efficiency, provide convenience, extend care to populations with limited access to transportation, and serve as a major influence on how nurses practice (Huston, 2013; Organisation for Economic Co-operation and Development, 2013). When designed and implemented to support nurses' work and workflow, technology can provide data transparency and offer a better work environment for nurses. As Dr. Pamela Cipriano has noted, work environments include conventional locations—hospitals, clinics, and patient homes—as well as virtual spaces, such as online discussion groups, email, interactive video, and virtual interaction (as cited in IOM, 2010a). Cipriano states that, ideally, technology eliminates redundancy and duplication of documentation; reduces errors; eliminates interruptions for missing supplies, equipment, and medications; and eases access to data, thereby allowing the nurse more time with the patient (as cited in IOM, 2010a). Perhaps, one of the most daunting challenges for nurses will be to retain the human element in practice. Other challenges include balancing cost with benefits, training the nursing workforce with a plan for sustainment, and ensuring the ethical use of technology (Huston, 2013).

Technology affects forensic nursing across all domains of practice, including patient care, coordination of care, and clinical and professional services. Although technology can enhance forensic nursing practice, it is also adversely used in the abuse, control, and harassment of patients/victims (e.g., sexual exploitation, intimate partner violence, child pornography). Forensic nurses must be cognizant that the same technologies used to promote forensic nursing care may have been used to inflict harm on the patient (e.g., camera, video equipment, digital recording devices).

Records and records storage: Forensic nurses must also be aware of technology and storage issues related to medical–forensic record retention policies and practices, including record storage requirements and destruction implications outside the normal, expected parameters for the medical record. The storage requirements for forensic nursing documentation should envisage secure criminal justice access to the medical–forensic record, the statutes of limitations for criminal and civil proceedings, the implications for cold cases, and future technological advances in the sciences.

Healthcare services delivery and coordination: Technology—such as telehealth, telemedicine, wireless transmission of secured data, and digital transmission of patient data across tablets or mobile devices—has forever changed the delivery and coordination of healthcare services. Advances in technology that influence nursing practice and patient care also affect forensic nursing practice. Forensic nurses are expected to evaluate and integrate new technologies for delivering forensic healthcare services. At times, this evaluation may comprise a critical appraisal of whether a new technology enhances or impedes patient/victim-centered care.

Limitations and implications of technology: Forensic nurses must remain diligent in reviewing and critically assessing the literature related to new technologies (or new applications of existing technologies) to understand the limitations of use or the interpretation of results. In addition, forensic nurses are expected to be aware of any legal regulations regarding the use of technology, including, but not limited to, licensure across state lines and the secure use and maintenance of electronic medical records (e.g., Health Insurance Portability and Accountability Act of 1996, Pub. L. No. 104-191, 110 Stat. 1936; Health Information Technology for Economic and Clinical Health Act of 2009, Pub. L. No. 111-5, 123 Stat. 226).

Advances in forensic science technology and techniques (e.g., Y-STR, next-generation sequencing) directly affect the forensic nurse regarding sample collection, preservation, and timeframes for providing medical–forensic examinations. In addition, forensic nurses must be aware of how perpetrators may use technology to inflict harm. For example, technology can be used to identify, locate, track, access, control, or intimidate patients/victims. Lastly, technology offers additional options for victims of violence, such as mobile applications for documenting injury, reporting crimes, and locating services. Forensic nurses are expected to incorporate the needs, expectations, and implications of an ever-evolving, technologically savvy society.

Availability and Access to Forensic Nursing Services

Forensic nurses serve widely diverse populations of patients affected by violence, including populations "never-served" by the healthcare community until the health and legal systems intersect. Due to the recognized need for forensic health care for populations that have experienced specific forms of violence involving unique dynamics, forensic nurses provide care to specific populations such as the following:

- Older adults

- Persons who are victims of human trafficking

- Persons seeking political asylum who have been tortured and/or experienced violence in their country of origin, during transit, or in internment facilities

- Persons affected by gang-related violence

- Persons who are stalked

- Persons who are affected by systematic violence

- Women and girls who have experienced female genital mutilation

- Persons who have been victimized through the use of technology (e.g., child pornography, cyberbullying, stalking)

- Persons who have been subjected to human rights violations (e.g., torture, government-sanctioned violence, mass killing and associated exhumations)

- Persons accused or suspected, but not yet convicted, of crimes

- Persons convicted of crimes

Forensic nurses serve as change agents and engage in specialized education and cross-sector training to identify and meet the unique needs of these specific forensic patients. Forensic nurses are critical to effecting change and increasing availability and access to services for all persons affected by violence. Collaborating with individuals, communities, organizations, and governments that support the development of the forensic nursing role brings international recognition to the forensic nursing specialty. The specialty knowledge—with acceptance and understanding of the scope and standards of practice—will continue to improve the response to patients across the globe who require forensic health care in multidisciplinary systems.

Forensic Nursing and Public Health: A Global Focus

Forensic nursing and public health nursing are inextricably linked, particularly in the primary, secondary, and tertiary care regarding intentional and unintentional injury involving individuals, families, groups, communities, and populations. Future master's and doctoral curricula internationally will use the graduate public health nursing competencies (QUAD Council, 2011) as a basis for forensic care of populations served by forensic nurses. Incorporation of public health concepts is essential in master's and doctoral education competencies (AACN, 2006). In addition, an emphasis on prevention, health promotion, formative and summative program evaluation, and sustainability helps to meet the pressing needs in patient populations at risk for injury and death from violence and trauma. The forensic nurse influences policy, practice, legislation, and trends when addressing issues of population-focused care related to intentional and unintentional injury, and death prevention and intervention. As a well-educated and respected professional, the forensic nurse links principles of public health and forensic sciences to forensic nursing practice, resulting in a broadening foundation for evaluating and managing injury and preventable death in populations worldwide. (For more on the international aspects of forensic nursing, see pages 32–33.)

Forensic Nursing Research and Its Global Influence

Forming the foundation for evidence-based practice, research supports the forensic nurse's role. Forensic nursing research is expected to accelerate; forensic nurse clinicians, educators, and researchers require and produce scientific evidence to support their growing practices. Informatics provides the conduit for the rapid dissemination of forensic nursing research (O'Carroll & Public Health Informatics Competencies Working Group, 2002). Forensic nursing research influences government policy, legislation, and action as the scientific base increases and the forensic nursing community expands its graduate education, experience, and credentialing processes. The international interprofessional community should increasingly acknowledge forensic nurses as valuable team members in addressing issues around persons and populations who have experienced violence, trauma, and abuse.

Summary of the Scope of Forensic Nursing Practice

Forensic nurses remain one of the most diverse groups of clinicians in the nursing profession with respect to patient populations served, practice settings, and forensic and healthcare services provided. The forensic nurse seeks educational opportunities to enhance her or his ability to better serve the ever-growing forensic healthcare needs of patients and populations. In addition, the forensic nurse must maintain and foster strong interprofessional relationships to meet the comprehensive forensic healthcare needs of patients and to ensure that patient-centered and trauma-informed care is provided throughout the continuum of care. Acts of violence, trauma, disaster, and crime-related deaths do not occur in a vacuum. Forensic nurses are acutely aware of how these acts directly and indirectly affect patients, families, communities, systems, and all of society. Forensic nurses continue to respond to the public health issue of violence across the life span through evidence-based and research-informed primary, secondary, and tertiary forensic nursing interventions.

Standards of Forensic Nursing Practice

Significance of Standards

The Standards of Forensic Nursing Practice are authoritative statements of the duties that all forensic nurses—regardless of role, population, or subspecialty focus—are expected to perform competently. The standards published herein may be used as evidence of the standard of care, with the understanding that application of the standards is context dependent. The standards are subject to change with the dynamics of the nursing profession and the specialty of forensic nursing, as new patterns of professional practice are developed and accepted by the profession and the public. In addition, specific conditions and clinical circumstances may affect the application of the standards at a given time (e.g., during a natural disaster or epidemic). The standards are subject to formal, periodic review and revision.

The competencies that accompany each standard may demonstrate compliance with the corresponding standard. The list of competencies is not exhaustive. Whether a particular standard or competency applies depends upon the circumstances. The competencies presented for the forensic nurse level are applicable to *all* forensic nurses. Standards may include additional competencies delineated for the APRNs specializing in forensic nursing.

Standards of Practice
for Forensic Nurses

Standard 1. Assessment

The forensic nurse collects pertinent data and information relative to the patient's health, death, or the situation.

Competencies

The forensic nurse:

▶ Collects pertinent data, including but not limited to demographics; social determinants of health; health disparities; and physical, functional, psychosocial, emotional, cognitive, sexual, cultural, age-related, environmental, spiritual/transpersonal, clinical-forensic, and economic assessments in a systematic, ongoing process with compassion and respect for the inherent dignity, worth, and unique attributes of every person.

▶ Collects data of physical and behavioral findings in a systematic and ongoing process to provide nursing care to patients while identifying the implications of those findings.

▶ Recognizes the importance of the assessment parameters identified by the WHO; the U.S. Department of Health and Human Services, as with its Healthy People 2020 initiative (DHHS, 2015); or other organizations that influence nursing practice.

▶ Integrates knowledge from global and environmental factors into the assessment process.

▶ Elicits the patient's values, preferences, expressed and unexpressed needs, and knowledge of the medical–forensic healthcare situation.

▶ Recognizes the impact of her or his personal attitudes, values, and beliefs on the assessment process.

- ▶ Identifies barriers to effective communication based on psychosocial, literacy, financial, and cultural considerations.

- ▶ Assesses the impact of family dynamics on the patient's health and wellness.

- ▶ Engages the patient and other interprofessional team members in holistic, culturally sensitive, and developmentally appropriate data collection.

- ▶ Prioritizes data collection based on the patient's immediate condition, anticipated needs of the patient or situation, and preservation of samples with potential evidentiary value.

- ▶ Uses evidence-based assessment techniques, instruments, tools, available data, information, and knowledge relevant to the situation to identify patterns and variances.

- ▶ Uses analytical models and problem-solving tools in forensic nursing practice.

- ▶ Applies ethical, legal, and privacy guidelines and policies to the collection, maintenance, use, and dissemination of data and information.

- ▶ Recognizes the patient as the authority of his or her health by honoring care preferences.

- ▶ Documents relevant data accurately and in a manner that is accessible to the interprofessional team members as appropriate.

- ▶ Assesses the effect of interactions among individuals, family, group, community, and social systems on health, illness, safety, violence, trauma, and preventable death across the life span.

- ▶ Synthesizes the results and information leading to clinical understanding.

Additional competencies for the advanced practice registered nurse specializing in forensic nursing

In addition to the competencies of the forensic nurse, the advanced practice registered nurse specializing in forensic nursing:

- ▶ Initiates and interprets diagnostic tests and procedures that are relevant to the patient's current status and forensic nursing practice.

- ▶ Uses advanced assessment, knowledge, and skills to maintain, enhance, or improve health and social conditions.

Standard 2. Diagnosis

The forensic nurse analyzes assessment data to determine actual or potential diagnoses, problems, and issues.

Competencies

The forensic nurse:

- ▶ Identifies actual or potential risks to the patient's health and safety or barriers to health, which may include but are not limited to interpersonal, systematic, cultural, or environmental circumstances.

- ▶ Identifies clinical findings while recognizing normal and abnormal developmental and physical variations of the patient.

- ▶ Uses assessment data, standardized classification systems, technology, and clinical decision support tools to articulate actual or potential diagnoses, problems, and issues.

- ▶ Verifies the diagnoses, problems, and issues with the individual, family, group, community, population, and interprofessional colleagues.

- ▶ Prioritizes diagnoses, problems, and issues based on mutually established goals to meet the needs of the patient across the health–illness continuum.

- ▶ Collaboratively assists within the healthcare team in the formulation of a differential diagnosis based on the assessment, history, physical examination, and diagnostic test results.

- ▶ Documents diagnoses, problems, and issues in a manner that facilitates the determination of the expected outcomes and plan.

Additional competencies for the advanced practice registered nurse specializing in forensic nursing

In addition to the competencies of the forensic nurse, the advanced practice registered nurse specializing in forensic nursing:

- ▶ Utilizes complex data and information obtained during the medical–forensic history, examination, diagnostic procedures, and review of medical–forensic documents in identifying diagnoses.

- ▶ Formulates a differential diagnosis based on the assessment, history, physical examination, and diagnostic test results.

- ▶ Systematically compares and contrasts clinical findings with normal and abnormal variations and developmental status in formulating a differential diagnosis.

- ▶ Assists staff in developing and maintaining competence in the diagnostic process.

- ▶ Uses information and communication technologies to analyze diagnostic practice patterns of nurses and other members of the interprofessional healthcare and multidisciplinary team.

- ▶ Employs aggregate-level data to articulate diagnoses, problems, and issues incurred by patients accessing medical–forensic healthcare services and organizational systems.

Standard 3. Outcomes Identification

The forensic nurse identifies expected outcomes for a plan individualized to the patient or the situation.

Competencies

The forensic nurse and the advanced practice registered nurse specializing in forensic nursing:

▶ Engage the patient, interprofessional team, and others in partnership to identify expected outcomes.

▶ Formulate culturally sensitive, developmentally appropriate expected outcomes derived from assessments, patient preferences, and diagnoses.

▶ Use clinical expertise and current evidence-based practice to identify health risks, benefits, costs, and/or the expected trajectory of the condition.

▶ Collaborate with the patient and family to define expected outcomes integrating the patient's developmental level, culture, values, and ethical considerations, including those associated with risks, benefits and costs, medical–forensic factors, clinical expertise, and current scientific evidence.

▶ Generate a timeframe for the attainment of expected outcomes.

▶ Develop expected outcomes that facilitate coordination of care and access to resources necessary for healing and patient safety.

▶ Modify expected outcomes based on the evaluation of the status of the patient and situation.

▶ Identify expected outcomes that incorporate cost and clinical effectiveness, best practices, and reflect trauma-informed patient care.

▶ Define expected outcomes that align with the outcomes identified by members of the interprofessional team.

▶ Differentiate outcomes that require care process interventions from those that require system-level actions.

▶ Advocate for outcomes that reflect the patient's developmental level, culture, values, and ethical concerns.

► Identify expected outcomes to effect systems changes to impact patient care.

► Evaluate the actual outcomes in relation to expected outcomes, safety, and quality standards.

► Document expected outcomes as measurable goals.

Standard 4. Planning

The forensic nurse develops a plan that prescribes strategies to attain expected, measurable outcomes.

Competencies

The forensic nurse:

▶ Develops an individualized, developmentally appropriate, holistic, evidence-based plan in partnership with the patient, family, interprofessional team, and others as appropriate.

▶ Establishes the plan priorities with the patient, family, interprofessional team, and others as appropriate.

▶ Advocates for responsible and appropriate use of interventions to minimize unwarranted or unwanted treatment and/or patient suffering.

▶ Prioritizes elements of the plan based on the assessment of the patient's level of risk and safety needs.

▶ Includes evidence-based strategies in the plan to address each of the identified diagnoses, problems, or issues. These strategies may include but are not limited to:

   ▶ Promotion and restoration of health;

   ▶ Prevention of illness, injury, disease, and death;

   ▶ Facilitation of healing;

   ▶ Alleviation of suffering; and

   ▶ Applicable supportive care.

▶ Incorporates an implementation pathway that describes steps and milestones.

▶ Considers the potential short- and long-term effects of violence and trauma across the life span for the patient, family, and community.

▶ Identifies cost and economic implications of the plan on the patient, family, caregivers, and other affected parties.

▶ Develops a plan that reflects compliance with current statutes, rules and regulations, and standards.

- Modifies the plan according to the ongoing assessment of the patient's response and other outcome indicators.

- Documents the plan using standardized language or recognized terminology.

- Actively participates in the development and continuous improvement of systems that support the planning process.

- Contributes to the design and development of interprofessional processes to address the identified diagnoses, problems, or issues.

- Designs innovative forensic nursing practices based on clinical practice experience, scientific advances, and research.

- Contributes to the development, evaluation, and continuous improvement of organizational systems that support the planning process.

Additional competencies for the advanced practice registered nurse specializing in forensic nursing

In addition to the competencies of the forensic nurse, the advanced practice registered nurse specializing in forensic nursing:

- Designs strategies and tactics to meet the multifaceted and complex needs of patients and medical–forensic situations.

- Leads the design and development of interprofessional processes to address the identified diagnoses, problems, or issues.

Standard 5. Implementation

The forensic nurse implements the identified plan.

Competencies

The forensic nurse:

▶ Partners with the patient and/or family to implement the plan in a safe, developmentally appropriate, effective, efficient, timely, patient-centered, and equitable manner (IOM, 2010b).

▶ Integrates interprofessional team members in implementation of the plan through collaboration and communication across the continuum of care.

▶ Demonstrates caring behaviors to develop therapeutic relationships.

▶ Provides culturally congruent, developmentally appropriate, holistic care that focuses on the patient and addresses and advocates for the needs of diverse populations across the life span.

▶ Uses evidence-based interventions and strategies to achieve the mutually identified goals and outcomes specific to the problem or needs.

▶ Integrates critical thinking and technology solutions in implementing the nursing process to collect, measure, record, retrieve, trend, and analyze data and information so as to enhance nursing practice and patient outcomes.

▶ Delegates according to the health, safety, and welfare of the patient, considering the circumstance, person, task, direction or communication, supervision, and evaluation, as well as the state nurse practice act regulations, the institution, and regulatory entities while maintaining accountability for care.

▶ Documents implementation and any modifications, including changes or omissions, of the identified plan.

▶ Uses systems, organizations, and community resources to lead effective change and implement the plan.

▶ Applies quality principles while articulating methods, tools, performance measures, and standards as they relate to implementation of the plan.

- Leads interprofessional teams to communicate, collaborate, and consult effectively.

- Demonstrates leadership skills that emphasize ethical and critical decision-making, effective working relationships, and a systems perspective.

- Serves as a consultant to provide additional insight and potential solutions.

- Provides clinical consultation for patients and professionals related to complex clinical cases to improve forensic nursing care and patient outcomes.

Additional competencies for the advanced practice registered nurse specializing in forensic nursing

In addition to the competencies of the forensic nurse, the advanced practice registered nurse specializing in forensic nursing:

- Uses prescriptive authority, procedures, referrals, treatments, and therapies in accordance with state and federal laws and regulations.

- Prescribes traditional and integrative evidence-based treatments, therapies, and procedures that are compatible with the patient's cultural preferences and norms.

- Prescribes evidence-based pharmacologic agents and treatments according to clinical indicators and results of diagnostic and laboratory tests.

- Translates evidence and research into practice.

- Uses theory-driven approaches to effect organizational or systems change.

Standard 5A. Coordination of Care

The forensic nurse coordinates care delivery.

Competencies

The forensic nurse:

▶ Organizes the components of the plan.

▶ Collaborates with the patient and/or family to help manage health care based on mutually agreed-upon outcomes.

▶ Manages the patient's care to reach mutually agreed-upon outcomes.

▶ Engages patients in self-care to achieve preferred goals for quality of life.

▶ Assists the patient and/or family to identify options for care.

▶ Communicates with the patient, the interprofessional team, and community-based resources to effect safe transitions and continuity of care.

▶ Advocates for delivery of dignified and holistic care by the interprofessional team.

▶ Provides leadership in the coordination of interprofessional health care for integrated delivery of patient services to achieve safe, effective, efficient, timely, developmentally appropriate, patient-centered, and equitable care (IOM, 2010b).

▶ Identifies system and community resources that enhance delivery of care and referrals for patients across continuums.

▶ Provides leadership in coordination of medical–forensic care delivery with the interprofessional team.

▶ Documents the coordination of care.

Additional competencies for the advanced practice registered nurse specializing in forensic nursing

In addition to the competencies of the forensic nurse, the advanced practice registered nurse specializing in forensic nursing:

▶ Synthesizes data and information to prescribe and provide necessary system and community support measures, including modifications of environments.

▶ Provides leadership in coordination of medical–forensic care as part of the interprofessional healthcare team to deliver integrated care for patients across the life span.

Standard 5B. Health Teaching and Health Promotion
The forensic nurse employs strategies to promote health and a safe environment.

Competencies

The forensic nurse:

- ▶ Provides opportunities for the patient to identify needed healthcare promotion, disease prevention, and self-management topics.

- ▶ Uses health promotion and health teaching methods in collaboration with the patient's values, beliefs, health practices, developmental level, learning needs, readiness and ability to learn, language preference, spirituality, culture, and socioeconomic status.

- ▶ Uses feedback and evaluations from the patient to determine the effectiveness of the employed strategies.

- ▶ Uses technologies to communicate health promotion, disease prevention, and preventative death information to the patient.

- ▶ Provides patients with information about intended effects and potential adverse effects of the plan of care.

- ▶ Engages patient alliance and advocacy groups in health teaching and health promotion activities for patients.

- ▶ Provides anticipatory guidance to patients to promote health and prevent or reduce the risk of negative health outcomes, violence, trauma, and related deaths across the life span.

Additional competencies for the advanced practice registered nurse specializing in forensic nursing
In addition to the competencies of the forensic nurse, the advanced practice registered nurse specializing in forensic nursing:

- ▶ Synthesizes empirical evidence on risk behaviors, gender roles, learning theories, behavioral change theories, motivational theories, translational theories for evidence-based practice, epidemiology, and other related theories and frameworks when designing health education information and programs.

▶ Evaluates health information resources for applicability, cultural and developmental appropriateness, accuracy, readability, and comprehensibility to develop quality health information resources for the patient population served.

Standard 6. Evaluation

The forensic nurse evaluates progress toward attainment of goals and outcomes.

Competencies

The forensic nurse:

▶ Conducts a holistic, systematic, ongoing, and criterion-based evaluation of the goals and outcomes in relation to the structure, processes, and timeline prescribed in the plan.

▶ Collaborates in the evaluation process with the patient and others involved in the care or situation.

▶ Determines, in partnership with the patient and other stakeholders, the patient-centeredness, effectiveness, efficiency, safety, timeliness, and equitability (IOM, 2001) of the strategies in relation to the responses to the plan and attainment of outcomes. Other defined criteria (e.g., Quality and Safety Education for Nurses) may be used as well.

▶ Uses ongoing assessment data to revise the diagnoses, outcomes, plan, and implementation strategies.

▶ Shares evaluation data and conclusions with the patient and other stakeholders in accordance with federal and state regulations.

▶ Documents the results of the evaluation.

Additional competencies for the advanced practice registered nurse specializing in forensic nursing

In addition to the competencies of the forensic nurse, the advanced practice registered nurse specializing in forensic nursing:

▶ Synthesizes evaluation data from the patient, community, population and/or institution to determine the effectiveness of the plan.

▶ Engages in a systematic evaluation process to revise the plan to enhance its effectiveness.

▶ Uses results of the evaluation to create, develop, or recommend process, policy, procedure, or protocol revisions when warranted.

Standards of Professional Performance for Forensic Nurses

Standard 7. Ethics

The forensic nurse practices ethically.

Competencies

The forensic nurse and the advanced practice registered nurse specializing in forensic nursing:

- ▶ Integrate the *Code of Ethics for Nurses with Interpretive Statements* (ANA, 2015a), IAFN's *Vision of Ethical Practice* (2008), the *ICN Code of Ethics for Nurses* (2012), and other comparable documents to guide forensic nursing practice and articulate the moral foundation of forensic nursing.

- ▶ Practice with compassion and respect for the inherent dignity, worth, and unique attributes of all people.

- ▶ Advocate for patients' rights to informed decision-making and self-determination.

- ▶ Seek guidance in situations where the rights of the individual conflict with public health guidelines.

- ▶ Endorse the understanding that the primary commitment is to the patient regardless of setting or situation.

- ▶ Maintain therapeutic relationships and professional boundaries.

- ▶ Advocate for the rights, health, and safety of the patient and others.

- ▶ Safeguard the privacy and confidentiality of patients, others, and their data and information within ethical, legal, and regulatory parameters.

- ▶ Demonstrate professional accountability and responsibility for nursing practice.

- ▶ Maintain competence through continued personal and professional development.

- ▶ Demonstrate commitment to self-reflection and self-care.

- ▶ Contribute to the establishment and maintenance of an ethical environment that is conducive to safe, quality health care.

- ▶ Advance the profession through scholarly inquiry, professional standards development, and the generation of policy.

- ▶ Collaborate with other health professionals and the public to protect human rights, promote health diplomacy, enhance cultural sensitivity and congruence, reduce health disparities, and promote equitable services for patients accessing forensic nursing services.

- ▶ Articulate nursing values to maintain personal integrity and the integrity of the profession.

- ▶ Integrate principles of social justice into forensic nursing practice and policy.

- ▶ Participate in interprofessional teams to assess and respond to ethical risk, benefits, and outcomes for patients.

Standard 8. Culturally Congruent Practice

The forensic nurse practices in a manner that is congruent with cultural diversity and inclusion principles.

Competencies

The forensic nurse:

▶ Demonstrates respect, equity, and empathy in actions and interactions with all patients.

▶ Participates in lifelong learning to understand cultural preferences, worldview, choices, and decision-making processes of diverse patient populations.

▶ Recognizes her or his own values, beliefs, and cultural heritage.

▶ Applies knowledge of variations in health beliefs, practices, and communication patterns in all forensic nursing practice activities.

▶ Identifies the stage of the patient's acculturation and accompanying patterns of needs and engagement.

▶ Considers the effects and impact of discrimination and oppression on practice and health within and among vulnerable cultural groups in the community specifically served and in the larger context of potential patients.

▶ Uses skills and tools that are created with input and appropriately vetted for the culture, literacy, and language of the population served.

▶ Communicates with appropriate language and behaviors, including the use of medical interpreters and translators in accordance with patient preferences.

▶ Identifies the cultural-specific meaning of interactions, terms, and content.

▶ Respects patient decisions based on age, developmental stage, tradition, belief and family influence, and stage of acculturation.

▶ Advocates for policies that promote health and prevent harm among culturally diverse, under-served, or under-represented patient populations.

▶ Promotes equal access to services, care, tests, interventions, health promotion programs, enrollment in research, education, and other opportunities.

▶ Educates nurse colleagues and other professionals about cultural similarities and differences of persons, families, groups, communities, and populations.

▶ Advances organizational policies, programs, services, and practices that reflect respect, equity, and values for diversity and inclusion.

▶ Engages patients, key stakeholders, and others in designing and establishing internal and external cross-cultural partnerships.

▶ Develops recruitment and retention strategies to achieve a multicultural workforce.

▶ Leads interprofessional teams to identify the cultural and language needs of the patient and populations served.

▶ Conducts research to improve health care, outreach, and healthcare outcomes for culturally diverse patient populations.

▶ Evaluates tools, instruments, and services provided to culturally diverse populations.

Additional competencies for the advanced practice registered nurse specializing in forensic nursing

In addition to the competencies of the forensic nurse, the advanced practice registered nurse specializing in forensic nursing:

▶ Promotes shared decision-making solutions in planning, prescribing, and evaluating processes when the patient's cultural preferences and norms may create incompatibility with evidence-based practice.

Standard 9. Communication

The forensic nurse communicates effectively in all areas of practice.

Competencies

The forensic nurse and the advanced practice registered nurse who specializes in forensic nursing:

- ▶ Assess their own communication skills and effectiveness.
- ▶ Demonstrate cultural empathy when communicating.
- ▶ Assess communication ability, health literacy, resources, and preferences of healthcare patients to inform the interprofessional team and others.
- ▶ Use appropriate language interpretation/translation resources to ensure effective communication.
- ▶ Incorporate appropriate alternative strategies to communicate effectively with patients who have visual, speech, language, or communication difficulties.
- ▶ Use developmentally appropriate communication styles and methods that demonstrate caring, respect, deep listening, authenticity, and trust.
- ▶ Convey accurate information.
- ▶ Maintain communication with the patient, family, interprofessional team, and others to facilitate safe transitions and continuity in care delivery.
- ▶ Contribute the forensic nursing perspective in interactions with others and in discussions with the interprofessional team.
- ▶ Expose care processes and decisions when they do not appear to be in the best interest of the patient.
- ▶ Disclose to the appropriate level their concerns related to potential or actual hazards and errors in care or the practice environment.
- ▶ Demonstrate continuous improvement of communication skills.
- ▶ Assume a leadership role in shaping or establishing environments that promote healthy communication.

Standard 10. Collaboration

The forensic nurse collaborates with the patient and other key stakeholders in the conduct of nursing practice.

Competencies

The forensic nurse and the advanced practice registered nurse specializing in forensic nursing:

▶ Identify the areas of expertise and contribution of other professionals and key stakeholders.

▶ Clearly articulate the forensic nurse's role and responsibilities within the team and to the patient.

▶ Use the unique and complementary abilities of all members of the team to optimize attainment of desired outcomes.

▶ Partner with the patient, family, and key stakeholders to advocate for and effect change, leading to positive outcomes and quality care.

▶ Use appropriate tools and techniques, including information systems and technologies, to facilitate discussion and team functions in a manner that protects dignity, respect, privacy, and confidentiality.

▶ Promote engagement through consensus building and conflict management.

▶ Use effective group dynamics and strategies to enhance team performance.

▶ Exhibit dignity and respect when interacting with others and giving and receiving feedback.

▶ Partner with all stakeholders to create, implement, and evaluate a comprehensive plan.

▶ Participate in interprofessional activities including but not limited to education, consultation, management, technological development, or research to enhance outcomes.

▶ Provide leadership for establishing, improving, and sustaining collaborative relationships to achieve safe, quality care for patients.

▶ Advance interprofessional plan-of-care documentation and communication, rationales for plan-of-care changes, and collaborative discussions to improve patient outcomes.

Standard 11. Leadership

The forensic nurse leads within the professional practice setting, the forensic nursing specialty, and nursing profession.

Competencies

The forensic nurse and the advanced practice forensic nurse specializing in forensic nursing specializing in forensic nursing:

- ▶ Contribute to the establishment of an environment that supports and maintains respect, trust, and dignity.

- ▶ Encourage innovation in practice and role performance to attain personal and professional plans, goals, and vision.

- ▶ Communicate ethically to manage change and address conflict.

- ▶ Mentor colleagues for the advancement of forensic nursing practice and the profession to enhance safe, quality health care.

- ▶ Retain accountability for delegated nursing care.

- ▶ Contribute to the evolution of the profession through participation in professional organizations.

- ▶ Influence policy to promote health.

- ▶ Influence decision-making bodies to improve the professional practice environment and patient outcomes.

- ▶ Enhance the effectiveness of the interprofessional team.

- ▶ Promote advanced practice nursing and role development by interpreting its role for patients and policy-makers.

- ▶ Model expert practice to interprofessional team members and patients.

- ▶ Mentor colleagues in the acquisition of clinical knowledge, skills, abilities, and judgment.

Standard 12. Education

The forensic nurse seeks knowledge and competence that reflects current forensic nursing practice and promotes futuristic thinking.

Competencies

The forensic nurse and the advanced practice registered nurse specializing in forensic nursing:

- ▶ Identify learning needs based on nursing knowledge and the various roles the nurse may assume.
- ▶ Participate in ongoing educational activities related to forensic nursing, interprofessional knowledge bases, and professional topics.
- ▶ Mentor forensic nurses who are new to their roles for the purpose of ensuring successful enculturation, orientation, and emotional support.
- ▶ Demonstrate a commitment to lifelong learning through self-reflection and inquiry for learning and personal growth.
- ▶ Seek experiences that reflect current practice to maintain and advance knowledge, skills, abilities, attitudes, and judgment in clinical practice or role performance.
- ▶ Acquire knowledge and skills relative to the role, population, specialty, setting, and global or local health situation.
- ▶ Participate in formal consultations or informal discussions to address issues in nursing practice as an application of education and knowledge.
- ▶ Identify modifications or accommodations needed in the delivery of education based on patient and family members' needs.
- ▶ Share educational findings, experiences, and ideas with peers.
- ▶ Support acculturation of forensic nurses who are new to their roles by role modeling, encouraging, and sharing pertinent information relative to optimal care delivery.
- ▶ Facilitate a work environment that supports the ongoing education of healthcare professionals.

- ▶ Maintains a professional portfolio that provides evidence of individual competence and lifelong learning.
- ▶ Develop and deliver academic curricula to nurses seeking undergraduate and advanced degrees in forensic nursing.

Standard 13. Evidence-Based Practice and Research

The forensic nurse integrates evidence and research findings into practice.

Competencies

The forensic nurse:

▶ Articulates the values of research and its application relative to the individual healthcare setting and practice.

▶ Identifies questions in the healthcare setting and practice that can be answered by forensic nursing research.

▶ Uses current evidence-based knowledge, including research findings, to guide practice.

▶ Incorporates evidence when initiating changes in nursing practice.

▶ Participates in the formulation of evidence-based practice through research.

▶ Promotes ethical principles of research in practice and the healthcare setting.

▶ Appraises nursing research for optimal application in practice and the healthcare setting.

▶ Shares peer-reviewed research findings with colleagues to integrate and advance knowledge in forensic nursing practice.

▶ Integrates research-based practice in all settings.

▶ Uses current healthcare research findings and other evidence to expand knowledge, skills, abilities, and judgment; enhance role performance; and increase knowledge of professional issues.

▶ Uses critical thinking skills to connect theory and research to practice.

▶ Integrates nursing research to improve quality in forensic nursing practice.

Additional competencies for the advanced practice registered nurse specializing in forensic nursing

In addition to the competencies of the forensic nurse, the advanced practice registered nurse specializing in forensic nursing:

▶ Contributes to forensic nursing knowledge by conducting or synthesizing research and other evidence that discovers, examines, and evaluates current practice, knowledge, theories, criteria, and creative approaches to improve healthcare outcomes, and shares findings with interdisciplinary colleagues and other forensic nurses.

▶ Encourages other forensic nurses to develop research skills and provides mentorship to others in this area.

▶ Performs rigorous critique of evidence that is derived from databases to generate meaningful evidence for forensic nursing practice.

▶ Advocates for the ethical conduct of research and translational scholarship with particular attention to the protection of the patient as a research participant.

▶ Promotes a climate of collaborative research and clinical inquiry.

▶ Disseminates research findings through activities such as presentations, publications, consultation, and journal clubs.

Standard 14. Quality of Practice

The forensic nurse contributes to quality nursing practice.

Competencies

The forensic nurse:

► Ensures that nursing practice is safe, effective, efficient, equitable, timely, and patient-centered (IOM, 1999, 2001).

► Identifies barriers and opportunities to improve forensic healthcare safety, effectiveness, efficiency, equitability, timeliness, and patient-centeredness.

► Recommends strategies to improve forensic nursing quality.

► Uses creativity and innovation to enhance forensic nursing care.

► Participates in quality improvement initiatives.

► Collects data to monitor the quality of forensic nursing practice.

► Contributes to efforts to improve forensic healthcare efficiency.

► Provides critical review and/or evaluation of policies, procedures, and guidelines to improve the quality of forensic health care.

► Engages in formal and informal peer review processes.

► Collaborates with the interprofessional team to implement quality improvement plans and interventions.

► Documents forensic nursing practice in a manner that supports quality and performance improvement initiatives.

► Achieves professional certification, when available.

► Incorporates evidence into forensic nursing practice to improve outcomes.

► Provides leadership in the design and implementation of quality improvement initiatives.

► Promotes a practice environment that supports evidence-based health care.

► Contributes to forensic nursing and interprofessional knowledge through scientific inquiry.

► Encourages professional or specialty certification.

- ▶ Engages in development, implementation, evaluation, and/or revision of policies, procedures, and guidelines to improve forensic healthcare quality.

- ▶ Uses data and information in system-level decision-making.

- ▶ Influences the organizational system to improve outcomes.

- ▶ Designs innovations to improve outcomes.

Additional competencies for the advanced practice registered nurse specializing in forensic nursing

In addition to the competencies for the forensic nurse, the advanced practice registered nurse specializing in forensic nursing:

- ▶ Analyzes trends in forensic healthcare quality data, including examination of cultural influences and factors.

- ▶ Engages in comparison evaluations of the effectiveness and efficacy of diagnostic tests, clinical procedures and therapies, and treatment plans in partnership with patients to optimize health and healthcare quality.

- ▶ Designs quality improvement studies, research, initiatives, and programs to improve health outcomes in diverse settings.

- ▶ Applies knowledge obtained from advanced preparation, as well as current research and evidence-based information, to clinical decision-making at the point of care to achieve optimal health outcomes.

- ▶ Uses available benchmarks to evaluate practice at the individual, departmental, or organizational level.

Standard 15. Professional Practice Evaluation

The forensic nurse evaluates one's own and others' nursing practice.

Competencies

The forensic nurse:

▶ Engages in self-reflection and self-evaluation of forensic nursing practice on a regular basis, identifying areas of strength as well as areas in which professional growth would be beneficial.

▶ Adheres to the guidance regarding professional practice as specified in *Nursing: Scope and Standards of Practice* (ANA, 2015b) and *Code of Ethics for Nurses with Interpretive Statements* (ANA, 2015a).

▶ Ensures forensic nursing practice is consistent with regulatory requirements pertaining to licensure, relevant statutes, rules, and regulations.

▶ Promotes incorporation of appropriate professional practice guidelines for the specific geographic region or practice area.

▶ Uses organizational policies and procedures as well as patient preference to guide forensic nursing professional practice.

▶ Influences organizational policies and procedures to promote interprofessional, evidence-based practice.

▶ Provides evidence for practice decisions and actions as part of the formal and informal evaluation processes.

▶ Seeks formal and informal feedback from healthcare patients, peers, colleagues, supervisors, and others regarding her or his practice.

▶ Provides peers and others with formal and informal constructive feedback regarding their practice or role performance.

▶ Takes action to achieve goals identified during the evaluation process.

Additional competencies for the advanced practice registered nurse specializing in forensic nursing

In addition to the competencies for the forensic nurse, the advanced practice registered nurse specializing in forensic nursing:

- ▶ Develops and/or identifies the tools used for evaluation of clinical forensic nursing practice.

- ▶ Engages in formal processes that involve feedback of forensic nursing practice from patients, peers, professional colleagues, and others.

- ▶ Assimilates the results of formal and informal evaluations into practice, policy, and protocols for enhancing the care of forensic patients.

Standard 16. Resource Utilization

The forensic nurse utilizes appropriate resources to plan, provide, and sustain evidence-based and research-informed nursing services that are safe, effective, and fiscally responsible.

Competencies

The forensic nurse:

▶ Assesses patient care needs and resources available to achieve desired outcomes.

▶ Assists the patient in factoring costs, risks, and benefits in decisions about care.

▶ Assists the patient in identifying and securing appropriate services to address needs across the healthcare continuum.

▶ Delegates in accordance with applicable legal and policy parameters.

▶ Identifies the impact of resource allocation on the potential for harm, complexity of the task, and desired outcomes.

▶ Advocates for resources that support and enhance forensic nursing practice.

▶ Integrates telehealth and mobile health technologies into practice to promote positive interactions between patients and forensic nurses and other healthcare providers.

▶ Uses organizational and community resources to implement inter-professional plans.

▶ Addresses discriminatory healthcare practices and the effect on resource allocation.

▶ Designs innovative solutions to use resources effectively and maintain quality.

▶ Creates evaluation strategies that address cost-effectiveness, cost/benefit, and efficiency factors associated with forensic nursing practice.

- ▶ Assumes complex and advanced leadership roles to initiate and guide change.

- ▶ Engages organizational and community resources to formulate and implement interprofessional plans.

Additional competencies for the advanced practice registered nurse specializing in forensic nursing

In addition to the competencies of the forensic nurse, the advanced practice registered nurse specializing in forensic nursing:

- ▶ Develops healthcare resources for patients, families, and communities that support and enhance forensic nursing practice.

- ▶ Formulates innovative solutions for patient care problems that use resources efficiently and effectively, and maintain quality.

- ▶ Designs evaluation processes to demonstrate effective resource utilization, avoid duplication of services, and promote patient safety and satisfaction while reducing cost.

Standard 17. Environmental Health

The forensic nurse practices in an environmentally safe and healthy manner.

Competencies

The forensic nurse and the advanced practice registered nurse specializing in forensic nursing:

▶ Promote a safe and healthy workplace and professional practice environment.

▶ Use environmental health concepts in practice.

▶ Assess the environment to identify risk factors.

▶ Reduce environmental health risks to self, colleagues, and patients.

▶ Communicate information about environmental health risks and exposure reduction strategies.

▶ Advocate for the safe, judicious, and appropriate use and disposal of products in health care.

▶ Incorporate technologies to promote safe practice environments.

▶ Use product or treatments consistent with evidence-based practice to reduce environmental threats.

▶ Participate in developing strategies to promote healthy communities and practice environments.

▶ Analyze the effect of social, political, and economic influences on the global environment and human health experience.

▶ Create partnerships that promote sustainable global environmental health policies and conditions that focus on prevention of hazards to people and the natural environment (ANA, 2007).

Glossary

Acculturation. The process by which an individual or group from one culture learns how to take on many of the behaviors, values, and ways of living of another culture. Few cultures become 100% acculturated to another cultural way of life. Cultures tend to be selective in what they choose to change and retain (Leininger & McFarland, 2002).

Accused. A person who has been formally charged with a crime and may be under arrest (freedom of movement limited) prior to a trial as opposed to a person of interest who is suspected but not charged with a crime.

Advanced practice registered nurses (APRN). "A nurse who has completed an accredited graduate level-education program preparing her or him for the role of certified nurse practitioner, certified registered nurse anesthetist, certified nurse midwife, or clinical nurse specialist; has passed a national certification examination that measures the APRN role and population-focused competencies; maintains continued competence as evidenced by recertification; and is licensed to practice as an APRN (Adapted from APRN JDG, 2008)" (ANA, 2015b, p. 85).

Assessment. "A systematic, dynamic process by which the registered nurse, through interaction with the patient, family, groups, communities, populations, and healthcare providers, collects and analyzes data. Assessment may include the following dimensions: physical, psychological, sociocultural, spiritual, cognitive, functional abilities, developmental, economic, and lifestyle" (ANA, 2015b, p. 85).

Autonomy (nurse). "The capacity of a nurse to determine her or his own actions through independent choice, including demonstration of competence, within the full scope of nursing practice" (ANA, 2015b, p. 85).

Autonomy (patient). The right of the patient to make choices about their health care and what is done to his or her body.

Caregiver. "A person who provides direct care for another, such as a child, dependent adult, the disabled, or the chronically ill" (ANA, 2015b, p. 5).

Caring. The moral ideal of nursing consisting of human-to-human attempts to protect, enhance, and preserve humanity and human dignity, integrity, and wholeness by assisting a person to find meaning in illness, suffering, pain, and existence (Watson, 2012).

Certification. "1. A process, often voluntary, by which individuals who have demonstrated the level of knowledge and skill required in the profession, occupation, role, or skill are identified to the public and other stakeholders. *2004 Standards Glossary.* 2. The voluntary process by which a non-governmental entity grants a time-limited recognition and use of a credential to an individual after verifying that he or she has met predetermined and standardized criteria. It is the vehicle that a profession or occupation uses to differentiate among its members, using standards, sometimes developed through a consensus driven process, based on existing legal and psychometric requirements. (This is the definition of 'professional certification' in the *2005 ICE Guide.*)" (Knapp, Fabrey, Rops, & McCurry, 2006).

Code of ethics (nursing). "A list of provisions that makes explicit the primary goals, values, and obligations of the nursing profession and expresses its values, duties, and commitments to the society of which it is a part. In the United States, nurses abide by and adhere to the *Code of Ethics for Nurses with Interpretive Statements*" (ANA, 2015b, p. 86).

Collaboration. "A professional healthcare partnership grounded in a reciprocal and respectful recognition and acceptance of: each partner's unique expertise, power, and sphere of influence and responsibilities; the commonality of goals; the mutual safeguarding of the legitimate interest of each party; and the advantages of such a relationship" (ANA, 2015b, p. 86).

Community. A social unit of any size that shares common values.

Competence. Successful performance at an expected level.

Competency. "An expected and measureable level of nursing performance that integrates knowledge, skills, abilities, and judgment, based on established scientific knowledge and expectations for nursing practice" (ANA, 2015b, p. 86).

Continuity of care. A process that involves patients, families, significant others, and multidisciplinary team members in the determination of a coordinated plan of care. This process facilitates the patient's transition between settings, healthcare providers, and multidisciplinary agencies and is based on changing needs and available resources in the community (adapted from ANA, 2015b, p. 86).

Cultural knowledge. "The concepts and language of an ethnic or social group used to describe their health-related values, beliefs, and traditional practices, as well as the etiologies of their conditions, preferred treatments, and any contraindications for treatments or pharmacologic agents interventions. Historical events, such as war-related migration, oppression, and structural discrimination are also included, when relevant" (ANA, 2015b, p. 86).

Cultural skills. "The integration of cultural knowledge and expertise into practice when assessing, communicating with, and providing care for members of a racial, ethnic, or social group" (ANA, 2015b, p. 86).

Criteria. Relevant, measurable indicators of the standards of practice and professional performance.

Data. Discrete entities that are described objectively without interpretation.

Death investigation. The scientific investigation of unlawful, unnatural, and suspicious deaths.

Diagnosis. "A clinical judgment about the [patient]'s response to actual or potential health conditions or needs. The diagnosis provides the basis for determination of a plan to achieve expected outcomes. Registered nurses utilize nursing and medical diagnoses depending upon educational and clinical preparation and legal authority" (ANA, 2015b, p. 86).

Domestic violence. (See Intimate partner violence.)

Environment. "The surrounding context, milieu, conditions, or atmosphere in which a registered nurse practices" (ANA, 2015b, p. 87).

Environmental health. "Aspects of human health, including quality of life, that are determined by physical, chemical, biological, social, and psychological problems in the environment. It also refers to the theory and practice of assessing, correcting, controlling, and preventing those factors in the environment that can potentially affect adversely the health of present and future generations" (ANA, 2015b, p. 87; Prüss-Ustün, Wolf, Corvalán, Bos, & Neira, 2016).

Evaluation. "The process of determining the progress toward [the] attainment of expected outcomes, including the effectiveness of care" (ANA, 2015b, p. 87).

Evidence. "Something (including testimony, documents, and tangible objects) that tends to prove or disprove the existence of an alleged fact; anything presented to the senses and offered to prove the existence or nonexistence of a fact" (Garner, 2014, p. 673).

Evidence-based practice. "Applying the best available research results (evidence) when making decisions about health care. Health care professionals who perform evidence-based practice use research evidence along with clinical expertise and patient preferences" (DHHS, Agency for Healthcare Research and Quality, n.d.).

Evidence-informed practice. Ensuring that health practice is guided by the best research and information available. Evidence may be qualitative or quantitative in nature and may derive from population health statistics, scientific journals and publications, evaluation reports, and locally collected data (Sawatzky-Dickson, 2010).

Expected outcomes. "End results that are measurable, desirable, and observable, and translate into observable behaviors" (ANA, 2015b, p. 68).

Expert witness. "A witness who qualified by knowledge, skill, experience, training, or education to provide a scientific, technical, or other specialized opinion about the evidence or a fact witness" (Garner, 2014, p. 1838).

Fact witness. "A witness who has firsthand knowledge of something based on the witness's perceptions through one or more of the five senses" (Garner, 2014, p. 1838).

Family. "Family of origin or significant others as identified by the [patient]" (ANA, 2015b, p. 87).

Forensic. Pertaining to law; for the purposes of this document, relating to the use of science or technology in the investigation and establishment of facts or evidence (*Merriam-Webster's*, 2008).

Forensic advanced practice registered nurse. A licensed registered nurse who has completed graduate or doctoral education with a specialization or emphasis in forensic nursing, and holds advanced practice registered nurse (APRN) credentials as a CNS, CNM, certified registered nurse anesthetist, or nurse practitioner.

Forensic nurse. An individual who is registered or licensed by a state, commonwealth, province, jurisdiction, territory, government, or other regulatory body to practice as a registered nurse and who has additional specialized education in forensic nursing.

Forensic nurse death investigator (FNDI). A forensic nurse who assists the coroner or medical examiner in determining the identity of the deceased, the time and place of death, and the cause and manner of death. An FNDI may also assist police at a crime scene or other investigative agencies in the course of their duties. The FNDI has a solid understanding of specimen collection, forensic photography, and legal process. An FNDI is skilled in pathology, physiology, observation, preservation, documentation of evidence, and knowledge of subsequent legal and criminal matters and testifying in court or quasi-judicial proceedings.

Forensic nursing. Practiced globally, forensic nursing is specialized nursing care that focuses on patient populations affected by violence and trauma—across the life span and in diverse practice settings. Forensic nursing includes education, prevention, and detection and treatment of the effects of violence in individuals, families, communities, and populations. Through leadership and interprofessional collaboration, the forensic nurse works to foster an understanding of the health effects, effective interventions, and prevention of violence and trauma. "The practice of nursing globally when health and legal systems intersect" (IAFN, 2017b).

Guidelines. Systematically developed statements that describe recommended actions based on available scientific evidence and expert opinion. Clinical guidelines describe a process of patient care management that has the potential of improving the quality of clinical and patient decision-making.

Health. "An experience that is often expressed in terms of wellness and illness, and may occur in the presence or absence of disease or injury" (ANA, 2015b, p. 87).

Healthcare providers. "Individuals with special expertise who provide healthcare services or assistance to patients. They may include nurses, physicians, psychologists, social workers, nutritionist/dietitians, and various therapists" (ANA, 2015b, p. 88).

Hearing. "A judicial session usu. open to the public, held for the purpose of deciding issues of fact or of law, sometimes with witnesses testifying" (Garner, 2014, p. 836).

Holistic care. "The integration of body–mind–emotion–spirit–sexual–cultural–social-energetic–environmental principles and modalities to promote health, increase well-being, and actualize human potential" (ANA, 2015b, p. 88).

Illness. "The subjective experience of discomfort, disharmony, or imbalance. Not synonymous with disease" (ANA, 2015b, p. 88).

Implementation. "Activities such as teaching, monitoring, providing, counseling, delegating, and coordinating" (ANA, 2015b, p. 88).

Implied consent. An agreement by a patient to allow disclosure of private health information in cases in which the patient has been informed about the information to be disclosed, the purpose of the disclosure, and his or her right to object to the disclosure, but has not done so. Implied consent is indicated by the behavior of an informed individual. It is essential that people with higher support and communication needs are given the time and assistance they need to give their consent on issues that involve them.

Information. "Data that are interpreted, organized, or structured" (ANA, 2015b, p. 88).

Informed consent. Voluntary agreement given by a person or a responsible proxy (e.g., a parent) for participation in a study, immunization program, or treatment regimen, after being informed of the purpose, methods, procedures, benefits, and risks. The essential criteria of informed consent are that the subject has both knowledge and comprehension, that consent is freely given without duress or undue influence, and that the right of withdrawal from the entity at any time is clearly communicated to the subject.

Injury. Any damage or harm done to or suffered by a person or thing that involves the bio-psycho-social, spiritual, or financial state of an individual, family, community, or system for which legal redress may be available. (*See also* Trauma.)

Interpersonal violence. Interpersonal violence occurs when one person uses power and control over another through physical, sexual, or emotional threats or actions, economic control, isolation, or other kinds of coercive behavior.

Interprofessional competencies. "Integrated enactment of knowledge, skills, and values/attitudes that define working together across the professions, with other health care workers, and with patients, along with families and communities, as appropriate to improve health outcomes in specific care contexts" (IECEP, 2011, p. 8).

Interprofessional team. "Reliant on the overlapping knowledge, skills, and abilities of each professional team member. This can drive synergistic effects by which outcomes are enhanced and become more comprehensive than a simple aggregation of the individual efforts of the team members" (ANA, 2015b, p. 88). (*See also* Multidisciplinary team.)

Intimate partner violence. Describes physical, sexual, or psychological harm by a current or former partner or spouse. This type of violence occurs among heterosexual or same-sex couples and does not require sexual intimacy.

Knowledge. Information that is synthesized so that relationships are identified and formalized.

Legal. Pertaining to the law; used for the purposes of this document as a broad term to describe criminal and civil justice systems and investigative disciplines.

Multidisciplinary team. "Reliant on the overlapping knowledge, skills, and abilities of each professional team member. This can drive synergistic effects, by which outcomes are enhanced and become more comprehensive than a simple aggregation of the individual efforts of the team members" (ANA, 2015b, p. 88). (*See also* Interprofessional team.)

Nursing. "The protection, promotion, and optimization of health and abilities, prevention of illness and injury, alleviation of suffering through the diagnosis and treatment of human response, and advocacy in the care of individuals, families, groups, communities, and populations" (ANA, 2015b, p. 88).

Nursing practice. "The collective professional activities of nurses characterized by the interrelations of human responses, theory application, nursing actions, and outcomes" (ANA, 2015b, p. 88).

Nursing process. "A critical thinking model used by nurses that comprises the integration of the singular, concurrent actions of these six components: assessment, diagnosis, identification of outcomes, planning, implementation, and evaluation" (ANA, 2015b, p. 88).

Offender. One who commits, executes, or performs a criminal act of any kind, has been deemed guilty in a court of law, and whose profiles and treatment modalities are integral to forensic nursing practice. One who has been deemed guilty in a court of law.

Patient. The person, client, family, group, community, or population, which comprises the focus of attention and to whom the registered nurse provides services as authorized by the state/provincial/jurisdictional regulatory bodies (adapted from ANA, 2015b, p. 88).

Patient-centered care. Health care that is closely congruent with and responsive to patients' wants, needs, and preferences.

Peer review. "A collegial, systematic, and periodic process by which registered nurses are held accountable for practice and that fosters the refinement of one's knowledge, skills, and decision-making at all levels and in all areas of practice" (ANA, 2015b, p. 89).

Plan. "A comprehensive outline of the components that need to be addressed to attain expected outcomes" (ANA, 2015b, p. 89).

Quality. "The degree to which health services for patients, families, groups, communities, or populations increase the likelihood of desired outcomes and are consistent with current professional knowledge" (ANA, 2015b, p. 89).

Registered nurse (RN). "An individual registered or licensed by a state, commonwealth, territory, government, or other regulatory body to practice as a registered nurse" (ANA, 2015b, p. 89).

Scope of Nursing Practice. "The description of the *who, what, where, when, why,* and *how* of nursing practice that addresses the range of nursing practice activities common to all registered nurses. When considered in conjunction with the Standards of Professional Nursing Practice and the Code of Ethics for Nurses, [the Scope of Nursing Practice] comprehensively describes the competent level of nursing common to all registered nurses" (ANA, 2015b, p. 89).

Sexual assault nurse examiner (SANE). A qualification for forensic nurses who have received special training to conduct sexual assault medical–forensic examinations for patients reporting a history of sexual assault.

Standards. "Authoritative statements defined and promoted by the profession by which the quality of practice, service, or education can be evaluated" (ANA, 2015b, p. 89).

Standards of Practice. Authoritative statements that "[d]escribe a competent level of nursing care as demonstrated by the nursing process" (ANA, 2015b, p. 89). (*See also* Nursing process.)

Standards of Professional Nursing Practice. "Authoritative statements of the duties that all registered nurses, regardless of role, population, or specialty, are expected to perform competently" (ANA, 2015b, p. 89).

Standards of Professional Performance. "Standards that describe a competent level of behavior in the professional role" (ANA, 2015b, p. 89). Registered nurses are accountable for their professional actions to themselves, their patients, their peers, and ultimately, society.

Suspect. A known person who is suspected of committing a crime but who has not been officially charged by the court and is not under arrest; a person of interest to the criminal legal system.

System. An assemblage of related elements that compose a unified whole, such as the legal and health systems, whose intersections provide the definitive context for forensic nursing, as well as the major systems in which forensic nurses practice:

- Health care (e.g., hospitals, surgery centers, community clinics)
- Investigative (e.g., medical examiner, coroner, law enforcement agencies, regulatory agencies)

- Criminal justice (e.g., prosecuting attorneys, public defenders, civil attorney offices)
- Correctional (e.g., jails, prisons, and detention centers)
- Public sector (e.g., military, local, state, provincial, and federal agencies)
- Educational (e.g., K–12 schools, colleges, universities)
- Private sector (e.g., industries, agencies, firms)
- International organizations (e.g., World Health Organization)

Testimony. "Evidence that a competent witness under oath or affirmation gives at trial or in an affidavit or deposition" (Garner, 2014, p. 1704).

Trauma. "Individual trauma results from an *event*, series of events, or set of circumstances that is *experienced* by an individual as physically or emotionally harmful or life threatening and that has lasting adverse *effects* on the individual's functioning and mental, physical, social, emotional, or spiritual well-being" (SAMHSA, 2014, p. 7). (*See also* Injury.)

Trauma-informed care/approach. Trauma-informed care is a treatment framework that involves understanding, recognizing, and responding to the effects of all types of trauma. "A program, organization, or system that is trauma-informed *realizes* the widespread impact of trauma and understands potential paths for recovery; *recognizes* the signs and symptoms of trauma in clients, families, staff, and others involved with the system; and *responds* by fully integrating knowledge about trauma into policies, procedures, and practices, and seeks to actively *resist re-traumatization*" (SAMHSA, 2014, p. 9).

Trial. "A formal judicial examination of evidence and determination of legal claims in an adversary proceeding"; "bench trial. A trial before a judge without a jury" (Garner, 2014, p. 1735); "jury trial. A trial in which the factual issues are determined by the jury, not by a judge" (Garner, 2014, p. 1736).

Victim. One who is acted upon and usually adversely affected by an outside incident. In forensic nursing, the victim may be the patient, the decedent, the perpetrator, the family, significant others, the suspect, the accused or falsely accused, the community, a population, a system, or the public in general.

Vision of Ethical Practice. An IAFN document describing the expectation that the forensic nurse aspires to the highest standards of ethical nursing practice (IAFN, 2008).

Vulnerable population. Includes persons who are economically disadvantaged, of racial and ethnic minority, uninsured, elderly, homeless; children of low-income families; and those with human immunodeficiency virus (HIV) and other chronic health conditions, including severe mental illness.

Wellness. "Integrated, congruent functioning aimed toward reaching one's highest potential" (Gaydos, 2005, p. 58).

Worldview. The way people look out at their universe and form a picture or value about their lives and the world around them (Leininger & McFarland, 2002). "Worldview includes one's relationship with nature, moral and ethical reasoning, social relationships, and magico-religious beliefs" (Purnell & Paulanka, 1998, p. 3).

References and Bibliography

All web sites accurate as of June 10, 2017.

American Association of Colleges of Nursing (AACN). (1995). *Position statement: Interdisciplinary education and practice.* http://www.aacn.nche.edu/publications/position/interdisciplinary-education-and-practice

American Association of Colleges of Nursing (AACN). (2006). *The essentials of doctoral education for advanced nursing practice.* Washington, DC: AACN. http://www.aacn.nche.edu/publications/position/DNPEssentials.pdf

American Association of Colleges of Nursing (AACN). (2008). *The essentials of baccalaureate education for professional nursing practice.* Washington, DC: AACN. http://www.aacn.nche.edu/education-resources/BaccEssentials08.pdf

American Board of Nursing Specialties (ABNS). (2016). *Summary Report, A National Convening—The Value of Certification: Building a Business Case for Certification,* Las Vegas, NV, March 3–5, 2016. Birmingham, AL: ABNS. http://www.nursingcertification.org/resources/documents/research/Value-of-Certification-Convening-Report-Final.pdf

American Nurses Association (ANA). (1991). *Position statement: Physical violence against women.* Washington, DC: ANA.

American Nurses Association (ANA). (2007). *ANA principles of environmental health for nursing practice with implementation strategies.* Silver Spring, MD: American Nurses Association. http://www.nursingworld.org/MainMenuCategories/WorkplaceSafety/Healthy-Nurse/ANAsPrinciplesofEnvironmentalHealthforNursingPractice.pdf

American Nurses Association (ANA). (2010a). *Nursing's social policy statement: The essence of the profession* (3rd ed.). Silver Spring, MD: Nursesbooks.org.

American Nurses Association (ANA). (2010b). *Recognition of a nursing specialty, approval of a specialty nursing scope of practice statement, and acknowledgement of specialty nursing standards of practice.* Silver Spring, MD: ANA. http://www.nursingworld.org/MainMenuCategories/Tools/3-S-Booklet.pdf

American Nurses Association (ANA). (2014). *ANA position statement: Professional role competence.* Silver Spring, MD: ANA. http://www.nursingworld.org/MainMenuCategories/ThePracticeofProfessionalNursing/NursingStandards/Professional-Role-Competence.html

American Nurses Association (ANA). (2015a). *Code of ethics for nurses with interpretive statements.* Silver Spring, MD: American Nurses Association.

American Nurses Association (ANA). (2015b). *Nursing: Scope and standards of practice* (3rd ed.). Silver Spring, MD: American Nurses Association.

American Nurses Association (ANA). (2016). *Leadership.* http://www.nursingworld.org/MainMenuCategories/ThePracticeofProfessionalNursing/Leadership

American Nurses Association (ANA) & International Association of Forensic Nurses (IAFN). (1997). *Scope and standards of forensic nursing practice.* Washington, DC: ANA.

American Nurses Association (ANA) & International Association of Forensic Nurses (IAFN) (2009). *Forensic nursing: Scope and standards of practice.* Silver Spring, MD: Nursesbooks.org.

ANA Leadership Institute. (2013). *Competency model.* Silver Spring, MD: American Nurses Association. https://learn.ana-nursingknowledge.org/template/ana/publications_pdf /leadershipInstitute_competency_model_brochure.pdf

APRN Joint Dialogue Group (APRN JDG). (2008). *Consensus model for APRN regulation: Licensure, accreditation, certification and education.* http://www.nursingworld.org /ConsensusModelforAPRN

Burgess, A. W., Berger, A. D., & Boersma, R. R. (2004). Forensic nursing: Investigating the career potential in this emerging graduate specialty. *American Journal of Nursing, 104*(3), 58–64.

Canadian Medical Association (CMA), Canadian Nurses Association (CNA), & Canadian Pharmacists Association (CPhA). (2003). *Joint position statement: Scopes of practice.* https:// www.cna-aiic.ca/~/media/cna/page-content/pdf-en/ps66_scopes_of_practice_june_2003_e .pdf?la=en

Canadian Nurses Association (CNA). (2008a). *Advanced nursing practice: A national framework.* Ottawa, ON: CNA. https://www.cna-aiic.ca/~/media/cna/page-content/pdf-en/anp _national_framework_e.pdf

Canadian Nurses Association (CNA). (2008b). *Code of ethics for registered nurses.* Ottawa, ON: CNA. http://www.nurses.ab.ca/content/dam/carna/pdfs/DocumentList/EndorsedPublications /RN_CNA_Ethics_2008.pdf

Canadian Nurses Association (CNA). (2015). *Framework for the practice of registered nurses in Canada* (2nd ed.). Ottawa, ON: CNA. http://www.cna-aiic.ca/~/media/cna/page-content /pdf-en/framework-for-the-pracice-of-registered-nurses-in-canada.pdf?la=en

Douglas, M. K., Rosenkoetter, M., Pacquiao, D. F., Callister, L. C., Milstead, J., Nardi, D., & Purnell, L. (2014). Guidelines for implementing culturally competent nursing care. *Journal of Transcultural Nursing, 25*(2), 109–121. doi: 10.1177/1043659614520998

Garner, B. A. (Ed.). (2014). *Black's law dictionary* (10th ed.). St. Paul, MN: Thomson Reuters.

Gaydos, H. L. B. (2005). The art of holistic nursing and the human health experience. In B. Dossey, C. Guzetta, & L. Keegan (Eds.), *Holistic nursing: A handbook for practice* (4th ed., pp. 57–76). Sudbury, MA: Jones and Bartlett Publishers.

Harris, C. (2013). Occupational injury and fatality investigations: The application of forensic nursing science. *Journal of Forensic Nursing, 9*(4), 193–199.

Harris, M., & Fallot, R. D. (Eds.). (2001). *Using trauma theory to design service systems.* San Francisco, CA: Jossey-Bass.

Hodges, B. D. (2010). A tea-steeping or i-doc model for medical education? *Academic Medicine: Competing Models of Competence Development, 85*(9), S34–S44. doi: 10.1097/ACM .0b013e3181f12f32

Humphreys, J., & Campbell, J. C. (Eds.). (2011). *Family violence and nursing practice* (2nd ed.). New York, NY: Springer Publishing Company.

Huston, C. (2013). The impact of emerging technology on nursing care: Warp speed ahead. *Online Journal of Issues in Nursing, 18*(2), Manuscript 1. http://www.nursingworld.org /MainMenuCategories/ANAMarketplace/ANAPeriodicals/OJIN/TableofContents/Vol-18 -2013/No2-May-2013/Impact-of-Emerging-Technology.html

Institute of Medicine (IOM). (1999). *To err is human: Building a safer health system.* Washington, DC: National Academies Press. http://nationalacademies.org/hmd/reports/1999/to-err -is-human-building-a-safer-health-system.aspx

Institute of Medicine (IOM). (2001). *Crossing the quality chasm: A new health system for the 21st century.* Washington, DC: National Academies Press. http://nationalacademies.org/hmd /reports/2001/crossing-the-quality-chasm-a-new-health-system-for-the-21st-century.aspx

Institute of Medicine (IOM). (2010a). *A summary of the October 2009 forum on the future of nursing: Acute care.* Washington, DC: National Academies Press.

Institute of Medicine (IOM). (2010b). *The future of nursing: Leading change, advancing health.* Washington, DC: National Academies Press. http://nationalacademies.org/hmd/reports /2010/the-future-of-nursing-leading-change-advancing-health.aspx

Institute of Medicine (IOM). (2011). *The future of nursing: Focus on education.* http://www .nationalacademies.org/hmd/Reports/2010/The-Future-of-Nursing-Leading-Change -Advancing-Health/Report-Brief-Education.aspx

International Association of Forensic Nurses (IAFN). (2004). *Core competencies for advanced practice forensic nursing.* http://c.ymcdn.com/sites/www.forensicnurses.org/resource/resmgr /Education/APN_Core_Curriculum_Document.pdf? hhSearchTerms=%22Core+and +competencies+and+advanced+and+practice+and+forensic+and+n%22

International Association of Forensic Nurses (IAFN). (2008). *Vision of ethical practice.* http:// www.forensicnurses.org/?page=VisionEthicalPract

International Association of Forensic Nurses (IAFN). (2013a). *Forensic nurse death investigator education guidelines.* Elkridge, MD: IAFN. http://www.forensicnurses.org/resource/resmgr /Education/Nurse_Death_Investigator_Edu.pdf

International Association of Forensic Nurses (IAFN). (2013b). *Intimate partner violence education guidelines.* Elkridge, MD: IAFN. http://www.forensicnurses.org/resource/resmgr/Education /Intimate_Partner_Violence_Nu.pdf

International Association of Forensic Nurses (IAFN). (2015). *Sexual assault nurse examiner (SANE) education guidelines.* Elkridge, MD: IAFN. https://iafn.site-ym.com/?2015EdGuidelines

International Association of Forensic Nurses (IAFN). (2017a). *History of the Association.* http://www.forensicnurses.org/?page=AboutUS

International Association of Forensic Nurses (IAFN). (2017b). *What is forensic nursing?* http://www.forensicnurses.org/?page=WhatisFN

International Council of Nurses (ICN). (2012). *ICN code of ethics for nurses.* Geneva, Switzerland: ICN. http://www.icn.ch/images/stories/documents/about/icncode_english.pdf

International Council of Nurses (ICN). (2013). *Position statement: Scope of nursing practice.* http://www.icn.ch/images/stories/documents/publications/position_statements/B07_Scope _Nsg_Practice.pdf

Interprofessional Education Collaborative Expert Panel (IECEP). (2011). *Core competencies for interprofessional collaborative practice: Report of an expert panel.* Washington, DC: Interprofessional Education Collaborative. http://www.aacn.nche.edu/education-resources /ipecreport.pdf

Knapp, J., Fabrey, L., Rops, M., & McCurry, N. (2006). *Basic guide to credentialing terminology.* Washington, DC: Institute for Credentialing Excellence.

Koop, C. E. (1986, February 26). *Public health and private ethics.* Paper presented to the Round Table on Science and Public Affairs at Duke University, Durham, NC. http://profiles.nlm.nih .gov/QQ/B/B/F/W/_/qqbbfw.pdf

Leininger, M., & McFarland, M. R. (2002). *Transcultural nursing. Concepts, theories, research & practices* (3rd ed.). New York, NY: McGraw-Hill, Inc.

Levine, J., & Johnson, J. (2014). An organizational competency validation strategy for registered nurses. *Journal for Nurses in Professional Development, 30*(2), 58–65. doi: 10.1097 /NND.0000000000000041

Lynch, V. A. (1990). *Clinical forensic nursing: A descriptive study in role development* (Unpublished master's thesis). University of Texas, Arlington, TX.

Lynch, V. A. (1991). Forensic nursing in the emergency department: A new role for the 1990s. *Critical Care Nursing Quarterly, 14*(3), 69–86.

Lynch, V. A., & Duval, J. B. (2011). *Forensic nursing science* (2nd ed.). St. Louis, MO: Elsevier/Mosby.

Mason, T., & Mercer, D. (1996). Forensic psychiatric nursing: Visions of social control. *Australian and New Zealand Journal of Mental Health Nursing, 5*(4), 153–162.

Melnyk, B. M., Gallagher-Ford, L., Long, L. E., & Fineout-Overholt, E. (2014). The establishment of evidence-based practice competencies for practicing registered nurses and advanced practice nurses in real-world clinical settings: Proficiencies to improve healthcare quality, reliability, patient outcomes, and costs. *Worldviews Evidence-Based Nursing, 11*(1), 5–15. doi: 10.1111/wvn.12021

Merriam-Webster's collegiate dictionary, 11th ed. (2008). Springfield, MA: Merriam-Webster, Inc.

National Nursing and Nursing Education Taskforce (N3ET). (2006). *A national specialisation framework for nursing and midwifery*. Melbourne, Australia: Health Workforce Australia. http://www.dhs.vic.gov.au/nnnet/downloads/recsp_framework.pdf

O'Carroll, P. W., & Public Health Informatics Competencies Working Group. (2002). *Informatics competencies for public health professionals*. Seattle, WA: Northwest Center for Public Health Practice, University of Washington School of Public Health and Community Medicine.

Organisation for Economic Co-operation and Development (OECD). (2013). *Health at a glance 2013: OECD indicators*. Paris, France: OECD Publishing. http://dx.doi.org/10.1787/health_glance-2013-en

Price, B., & Maguire, K. (Eds.). (2015). *Core curriculum for forensic nursing*. Philadelphia, PA: Lippincott Wolters Kluwer.

Prüss-Ustün, A., Wolf, J., Corvalán, C., Bos, R., & Neira, M. (2016). *Preventing disease through healthy environments: A global assessment of the burden of disease from environmental risks*. Geneva, Switzerland: World Health Organization. http://apps.who.int/iris/bitstream/10665/204585/1/9789241565196_eng.pdf?ua=1

Purnell, L. D., & Paulanka, B. J. (1998). *Transcultural health care: A culturally competent approach*. Philadelphia, PA: F. A. Davis Company.

QUAD Council. (2011). *Quad Council competencies for public health nurses*. http://www.achne.org/files/Quad%20Council/QuadCouncilCompetenciesforPublicHealthNurses.pdf

Sawatzky-Dickson, D. (2010). *Evidence-informed practice resource package*. Winnipeg, Manitoba: Winnipeg Regional Health Authority. http://www.wrha.mb.ca/osd/files/EIPResourcePkg.pdf

Schober, M., & Affara, F. A. (2006). *International Council of Nurses: Advanced nursing practice*. Malden, MA: Blackwell Publishing.

Shives, L. R. (2011). *Basic concepts of psychiatric–mental health nursing* (8th ed.). Philadelphia, PA: Lippincott, Williams, and Wilkins.

Speck, P. M. (2000). *Things you didn't learn in nursing school: Forensic nursing principles—WHEEL*. Paper presented to the Emergency Nurses Association, Chicago, IL.

Speck, P. M., & Peters, S. (1999). Forensic nursing: Where law and nursing intersect. *Advance for Nurse Practitioners, 11*(10).

Substance Abuse and Mental Health Services Administration (SAMHSA). (2014). *SAMHSA's concept of trauma and guidance for a trauma-informed approach*. HHS Publication No. (SMA) 14-4884. Rockville, MD: SAMHSA. https://store.samhsa.gov/shin/content//SMA14-4884/SMA14-4884.pdf

United Nations. (1948). *Universal declaration of human rights, General Assembly resolution 217A (III).* http://www.un.org/Overview/rights.html

U.S. Department of Health and Human Resources (DHHS), Agency for Healthcare Research and Quality (AHRQ). (n.d.). *Effective health care program: Glossary of terms.* http://effective healthcare.ahrq.gov/index.cfm/glossary-of-terms/?pageaction=showterm&termid=24

U.S. Department of Health and Human Resources (DHHS), Health Resources and Services Administration (HRSA). (2010). *The registered nurse population: Findings from the 2008 National Sample Survey of Registered Nurses.* Rockville, MD: DHHS. http://bhpr.hrsa.gov /healthworkforce/rnsurveys/rnsurveyfinal.pdf

U.S. Department of Health and Human Resources (DHHS), Health Resources and Services Administration (HRSA). (n.d.). *HRSA data warehouse: National Sample Survey of Registered Nurses data download—1977–2008.* http://datawarehouse.hrsa.gov/data/dataDownload /nssrndownload.aspx

U.S. Department of Health and Human Services (DHHS), Office of Disease Prevention and Health Promotion. (2016). *Healthy people 2020.* https://www.healthypeople.gov/

Vessier-Batchen, M. (2007). *Life after death: A comparison of coping and symptoms of complicated grief in survivors of homicide and suicide decedents* (Doctoral dissertation). Dissertation abstracts international. (68, 06).

Watson, J. (2012). *Human caring science: A theory of nursing* (2nd ed.). Sudbury, MA: Jones and Bartlett Learning.

Wooten, R. (2003). Applying the nursing process to death investigation. *Forensic Nurse, November/December,* 8.

Appendix A.
Resources

All web sites accurate as of June 10, 2017.

International Association of Forensic Nurses (IAFN). (2008). *Vision of ethical practice.* Elkridge, MD: IAFN. http://www.forensicnurses.org/?page=visionethicalpract

International Association of Forensic Nurses (IAFN). (2013). *Forensic nurse death investigator education guidelines.* Elkridge, MD: IAFN. http://www.forensicnurses.org/resource/resmgr /Education/Nurse_Death_Investigator_Edu.pdf

International Association of Forensic Nurses (IAFN). (2013). *Intimate partner violence education guidelines.* Elkridge, MD: IAFN. http://www.forensicnurses.org/resource/resmgr/Education /Intimate_Partner_Violence_Nu.pdf

International Association of Forensic Nurses (IAFN). (2015). *Sexual assault nurse examiner (SANE) education guidelines.* Elkridge, MD: IAFN. https://iafn.site-ym.com/?2015 EdGuidelines

International Association of Forensic Nurses (IAFN). (2016). *Non-fatal strangulation documentation toolkit.* Elkridge, MD: IAFN. https://c.ymcdn.com/sites/iafn.site-ym.com /resource/resmgr/resources/Strangulation_Documentation_.pdf

International Association of Forensic Nurses. (2017). *Making the argument for SANE* [Video infographic]. http://www.forensicnurses.org/?page=SANE365

International Association of Forensic Nurses. (2017). *Sexual assault forensic examiner technical assistance.* http://www.safeta.org/. [Supported by funding from the Office on Violence Against Women, U.S. Department of Justice.]

International Association of Forensic Nurses. (2017). *Tribal forensic healthcare.* http://www .tribalforensichealthcare.org/. [Supported by funding from the U.S. Indian Health Service].

International Association of Forensic Nurses (IAFN) & Seedworks Films. (2011). *Forensic nursing documentary trailer* [Video snapshot of the world of the forensic nurse]. https://www.youtube .com/watch?v=6ivGR-BtEjA

International Association of Forensic Nurses (IAFN) & Seedworks Films. (2012). *Forensic nursing documentary part one* [Video snapshot of the world of the sexual assault nurse examiner]. https://www.youtube.com/watch?v=-Cj56hGyxag&t=45s

International Association of Forensic Nurses (IAFN) & Seedworks Films. (2012). *Forensic nursing documentary part two* [Video snapshot of the world of the forensic nurse death investigator]. https://www.youtube.com/watch?v=rYvdb-x7L0o

International Association of Forensic Nurses (IAFN) & Seedworks Films. (2012). *Forensic nursing documentary part three* [Video snapshot of general clinical forensic nursing practice]. https://www.youtube.com/watch?v=j-bHzqB640U

U.S. Department of Justice, Office for Victims of Crime. (2016). *SANE program development and operation guide.* Washington, DC: Department of Justice. https://www.ovcttac.gov/saneguide/introduction/

Appendix B.
Forensic Nursing: Scope and Standards of Practice (2009)

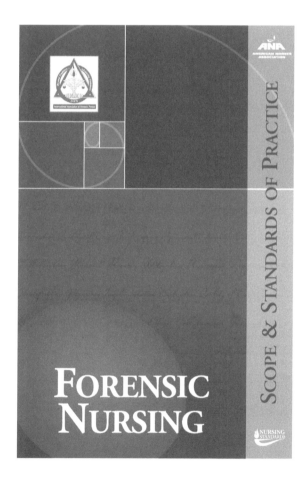

SCOPE & STANDARDS OF PRACTICE

FORENSIC NURSING

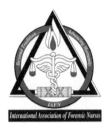

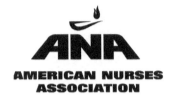

FORENSIC NURSING:
SCOPE AND STANDARDS
OF PRACTICE

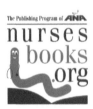

INTERNATIONAL ASSOCIATION OF FORENSIC NURSES

AMERICAN NURSES ASSOCIATION
SILVER SPRING, MARYLAND
2009

Library of Congress Cataloging-in-Publication data

International Association of Forensic Nurses.
Forensic nursing : scope and standards of practice / International Association of Forensic Nurses.
   p. ; cm.
Rev. ed. of: Scope and standards of forensic nursing practice / International Association of Forensic Nurses, American Nurses Association. c1997.
Includes bibliographical references and index.
ISBN-13: 978-1-55810-265-1 (pbk.)
ISBN-10: 1-55810-265-5 (pbk.)
   1. Forensic nursing—Standards. I. American Nurses Association.
II. International Association of Forensic Nurses. Scope and standards of forensic nursing practice. III. Title.
   [DNLM: 1. Forensic Nursing—standards—Guideline. 2. Professional Competence—standards—Guideline. WY 170 I61f 2009]

RA1155.I57 2009
614'.1—dc22   2009008708

The American Nurses Association (ANA) is a national professional association. This ANA publication—*Forensic Nursing: Scope and Standards of Practice*—reflects the thinking of the nursing profession on various issues and should be reviewed in conjunction with state board of nursing policies and practices. State law, rules, and regulations govern the practice of nursing, while *Forensic Nursing: Scope and Standards of Practice* guides nurses in the application of their professional skills and responsibilities.

The International Association of Forensic Nurses (IAFN) is an international membership organization comprised of forensic nurses working around the world and other professionals who support and complement the work of forensic nursing. The IAFN mission is to provide leadership in forensic nursing practice by developing, promoting, and disseminating information internationally about forensic nursing science. More at: http://www.forensicnurse.org

Published by Nursesbooks.org
The Publishing Program of ANA

American Nurses Association
8515 Georgia Avenue, Suite 400
Silver Spring, MD 20910-3492
1-800-274-4ANA
http://www.Nursesbooks.org/

The ANA is the only full-service professional organization representing the interests of the nation's 2.9 million registered nurses through its 53 constituent member nurses associations and its 24 specialty nursing and workforce advocacy affiliate organizations that currently connect to ANA as affiliates. The ANA advances the nursing profession by fostering high standards of nursing practice, promoting the rights of nurses in the workplace, projecting a positive and realistic view of nursing, and by lobbying the Congress and regulatory agencies on health care issues affecting nurses and the public.

Design: Scott Bell, Arlington, VA ~ Freedom by Design, Alexandria, VA ~ Stacy Maguire, Sterling, VA ~ *Editorial Management*: Eric Wurzbacher, ANA ~ *Copyediting*: Steven Jent, Denton, TX ~ *Proofreading*: Ashley Mason, Atlanta, GA ~ *Indexing*: Estalita Slivoskey, Havre de Grace, MD ~ *Composition*: House of Equations, Inc., Arden, NC ~ *Printing*: Linemark Printing, Upper Marlboro, MD

First printing May 2009.

ISBN-13: 978-1-55810-265-1   SAN: 851-3481   2.5M   05/09

ACKNOWLEDGMENTS

Forensic Nursing: Scope and Standards of Practice has taken five years to write. It was an International *volunteer* initiative, with four focus groups (2003–2005), one lengthy comment period (2004–2005), one Executive Committee Review (2007), one survey (2007), and several communications between ANA staff and Dr. Patricia M. Speck. The focus groups were held at the International Association of Forensic Nurses (IAFN) Scientific Assembly annually and attendees were invited to participate in the development of the body of work as content was changed and sections were completed (2003–2005). The document was presented to the membership of IAFN for comment after the major revisions were completed by posting online (2004–2005). The second comment period was from the Executive Committee of the Board of Directors (2007).

After the second submission to ANA, the definition of forensic nursing remained unclear to the non-forensic nurse reviewers. In response to the question "What is a forensic nurse, and what makes them unique and different from other nurse specialties?", a qualitative survey was developed by the primary authors and administered by IAFN, with an invitation to the membership to help define forensic nursing (2007–2008). Over 800 forensic nurses worldwide completed the survey.

From the survey's results, the primary authors created examples of forensic nursing practice and revised areas that ANA reviewers had identified as needing clarification. Furthermore, they integrated case scenarios in order to compare the intersecting roles of nursing and forensic nursing. The scenarios were added to the document. This part of the revision proved to be particularly arduous and time-consuming, but its complexity, magnitude, and potential impact demanded it. The primary authors also made additional recommended changes to clarify nursing language and hierarchy for the non-nurse reader. The final document was resubmitted to the two-step ANA review process in May 2008.

The primary authors wish to thank the IAFN Presidents (2003–2008) and the Boards of Directors (2003–2008) for their patience and gentle encouragement; the Focus Group attendees (2003–2006) for their content expertise and enthusiasm about this publication; the members of IAFN who continued to answer the primary authors' questions about the scope and detail of their practice each year as the development of this document progressed; the University of Tennessee Health Science Center College of Nursing, Office of Research and Grant Support (including Dr. Mona Wicks, Ms. Gail Spake, and Mr. Chris Peete for editorial support); and Dr. Carol Bickford and her staff at ANA for expertise, understanding, recommendations, and advice throughout the creation of this document.

Dr. Pat Speck

COMMITTEE TO WRITE *FORENSIC NURSING:* *SCOPE AND STANDARDS OF PRACTICE*

Chairperson (2003–2008):
Anita Hufft, PhD, RN

IAFN BOD Liaison:
Patricia M. Speck, DNSc, FNP-BC, FAAN, FAAFS, DF-IAFN, SANE-A, SANE-P
President, IAFN (2003–2004)
Immediate Past President, IAFN (2005–2006)
Past President, IAFN (2007–present)

Primary Authors:
Anita Hufft, PhD, RN

Patricia M. Speck, DNSc, FNP-BC, FAAN, FAAFS, DF-IAFN, SANE-A, SANE-P

Susan B. Patton, DNSc, APRN- BC, SANE-A, SANE-P

Focus Group Contributors:
Eileen Allen, MSN, RN, FN-CSA, SANE-A

Maggie Baker, PhD, RN

Kathleen Brown, PhD, CRNP

Ann W. Burgess, DNSc, APRN-BC

Cathy Carter-Snell, PhD(c), RN, SANE-A

Patricia Crane, PhD, MSN, WHNP, RNC

Donna Gaffney, DNSc, RN, FAAN, SANE-A

David Keepnews, PhD, JD, RN, FAAN

Arlene Kent-Wilkinson, PhD(c), RN

Louanne Lawson, PhD, RN, FAAN, DF-IAFN

Virginia Lynch, MSN, RN, FAAN, FAAFS

Barbara Moynihan, PhD, RN, APRN-BC

Cindy Peternelj-Taylor, MSc, BScN, RN

Julie Rosof-Williams, MSN, APRN-BC, SANE-A, SANE-P

L. Kathleen Sekula, PhD, APRN-BC

Deborah Shelton, PhD, RN, CNA BC

Daniel Sheridan, PhD, RN, FAAN

Sharon Stark, DNSc, RN APN-C

Deborah Travis, MN, RN, SANE-A, CNS

Melissa Vessier-Batchen, DNS, RN, CFN

Cathy Young, DNSc, APRN-BC

American Nurses Association (ANA) Staff
Carol J. Bickford, PhD, RN-BC – Content editor

Yvonne Humes, MSA – Project coordinator

Maureen E. Cones, Esq. – Legal counsel

CONTENTS

Appendix B. Forensic Nursing: Scope and Standards of Practice (2009)

SCOPE AND STANDARDS OF FORENSIC NURSING PRACTICE

Introduction

Forensic Nursing: Scope and Standards of Practice identifies the expectations for the role and practice of the forensic nurse. It builds on the first version of this material, *Scope and Standards of Forensic Nursing*, co-published in 1997 with the American Nurses Association (ANA) and the International Association of Forensic Nurses (IAFN). The entire updated statement of scope and standards of forensic nursing practice is meant to define and direct forensic nursing practice in all settings and across all roles. This complex and comprehensive consensus document has been developed with input from International Association of Forensic Nurses (IAFN) membership, among others, and uses the ANA framework and guide for scope and standards documents approved by the Congress on Nursing Practice and Economics (ANA, 2005).

Function of the Scope of Practice Statement

The scope of practice statement (pages 1–21) describes the "who", "what", "where", "when", "why" and "how" of nursing practice. Each of these questions must be sufficiently answered to provide a complete picture of the practice and its boundaries and membership. The depth and breadth in which individual registered nurses engage in the total scope of nursing practice is dependent upon education, experience, role, and the population served.

Function of Standards

The Standards, which are comprised of the standards of practice (pages 23–34) and the standards of professional performance (pages 35–48), are authoritative statements by which nurses practicing within the role, population, and specialty governed by this document (*Forensic Nursing: Scope and Standards of Practice*) and describe the duties that they are expected to competently perform. The Standards published herein may be utilized as evidence of the legal standard of care governing nurses practicing within the role, population, and specialty governed by this document. The Standards are subject to change with the dynamics of the nursing profession and as new patterns of professional practice are developed and accepted by the nursing profession and the public. In addition, specific conditions and clinical circumstances may also affect the application of the Standards at a given time; e.g., during a natural disaster. The Standards are subject to formal, periodic review and revision.

The measurement criteria that appear below each standard are not all-inclusive and do not establish the legal standard of care. Rather, the measurement criteria are specific, measurable elements that can be used by nursing professionals to measure professional performance. Nurses practicing within this particular role, population, and specialty can identify opportunities for development and improvement by evaluating performance on these elements.

Forensic Nursing's International Context

Dramatic changes in health care and the profession of nursing have occurred worldwide during the past decade. Ethical codes developed by various nursing organizations provide significant guidance for all nurses and for nursing practice in every setting (ANA, 2001, 2005; CNA, 2002; IAFN, 2006; ICN, 2006). Evolving professional and societal needs and expectations necessitate a statement to clarify the scope of practice for the nurse. Similarly, the demand for the credentialing of nurses in specialty practice mandates consistent and standardized processes for defining the focus and competencies of specialty practice (ANA, 2004, 2005).

The American Nurses Association has responded with updated versions of the three documents that provide the foundation of practice in the United States: the *Code of Ethics for Nurses with Interpretive Statements* (2001), *Nursing's Social Policy Statement, 2nd Edition* (2003), and *Nursing: Scope and Standards of Practice* (2004). The Canadian Nurses Association and the Canadian Federation of Nurses Unions have affirmed similar changes with the adoption of the *Joint Position Statement Scopes of Practice* (2006) and *Advanced Nursing Practice: A National Framework* (2008). Documents such as the Canadian Nurses Association's *Framework for the Practice of Registered Nurses in Canada* (2007), Australia's National Nursing & Nursing Education Taskforce's *A National Specialisation Framework for Nursing and Midwifery* (2006), ANA's *Nursing: Scope and Standards of Practice* (2004), and the International Council of Nurses' position statement *Scope of Nursing Practice* (2004) delineate the boundaries of professional nursing practice and provide a framework within which nursing specialties globally can establish role expectations across all settings, including practice, education, administration, and research. The organization and content of these documents, as well as the expansion and evolution of the nursing specialty internationally (Schober & Affara, 2006), have necessarily altered the format and content of the scope and standards of forensic nursing practice.

Forensic Nursing: Scope and Standards of Practice defines and comprehensively describes forensic nursing as a specialty and provides direction for further progress and recognition internationally. Recognized as a nursing specialty in 1995 by the ANA, forensic nursing represents the response of nurses to the rapidly changing healthcare environment and to the global challenges of caring for victims and perpetrators of intentional and unintentional injury.

The scope of forensic nursing practice exists within flexible boundaries across diverse settings and populations. Forensic nurses care for individuals, families, and communities whose status or care is, in part, determined by legal or forensic issues. These patients are encountered in a variety of settings including healthcare, educational, legal, legislative, and scientific systems.

The practice of all professional nurses now includes many of the concepts previously deemed unique to the forensic nursing specialty, including violence, prevention of injury, victimization, abuse, and exploitation. Today, nurses in any country, setting, or system are expected to plan for the care of a patient who has been injured through intentional or unintentional acts that involve violence and victimization.

As the body of knowledge and skill sets identified as unique to forensic nursing expands, so does the practice of forensic nursing. The specialty's scope statement and standards of practice are intended to serve as a foundation for legislation and regulation of forensic nursing, along with the development of institutional policies and procedures for those settings in which forensic nurses practice. Given rapid changes in healthcare trends and technologies, the standards in this document are intended to be dynamic and futuristic, allowing flexibility in response to emerging issues and practices of forensic nursing.

Additional Content

For a better appreciation of the historical and professional context underlying *Forensic Nursing: Scope and Standards of Practice*, the content of *Scope and Standards for Forensic Nurse* (1997) has been reproduced in Appendix A (starting on page 57) and is indexed with the current content of this edition. That 1997 publication was the immediate predecessor to this current edition. Its content is not current and is of historical significance only.

Scope of Forensic Nursing Practice

Function of the Scope of Practice Statement

The scope of practice statement (pages 1–21) describes the "who", "what", "where", "when", "why" and "how" of nursing practice. Each of these questions must be sufficiently answered to provide a complete picture of the practice and its boundaries and membership. The depth and breadth in which individual registered nurses engage in the total scope of nursing practice is dependent upon education, experience, role, and the population served.

Overview of Forensic Nursing

Forensic nursing is a multifaceted and complex practice specialty characterized by responsibilities, functions, roles, and skills that have been derived from general nursing practice, yet also developed in accordance with the distinctive practice environments and populations of forensic nursing. Forensic nursing practice, concerned primarily with the victims and perpetrators of trauma, their families, communities, and the systems that respond to them, may include but is not limited to:

- Assessment, diagnosis, planning, implementation, evaluation of, and scientific inquiry about human, program, and system responses to injury and interventions following injury to individuals, communities, cultures, and environments.

- Identification of the pathology of intentional or unintentional injury in those living and deceased.

- Collection and analysis of evidentiary material.

- Participation in the generation, dissemination, and utilization of evidence-based research in forensic nursing practice delivered to patients, communities, and systems.

- Utilization of formative and summative evaluation processes in forensic nursing roles and environments internationally.

- Administration, organization, and coordination of the forensic nursing role in programs, systems, and environments where forensic nurses practice.

- Involvement and influence in both internal and external systems where professional and societal regulation of forensic nursing practice impacts public health and safety.

- Development and support of local, regional, and global policy and public health as it relates to injury and the prevention of injury in a variety of cultures and communities.

- Promotion of and accountability to the ethical paradigms within forensic nursing.

- Development and implementation of professional and community education programs of interest to forensic nurses that address prevention and interventions in primary, secondary, and tertiary settings.

- Development and promotion of the interprofessional collaboration between the forensic nurse and others in all roles and practice environments.

Definition and Evolution of Forensic Nursing

The original definition of forensic nursing was "the application of nursing process to public or legal proceedings" (Lynch, 1990). The foundation of forensic nursing practice is the rich bio-psycho-social-spiritual education of registered nurses, and uses the nursing process to diagnose and treat victims and perpetrators of trauma, their families, communities, and the systems that respond to them.

Forensic nursing focuses on the identification, management, and prevention of intentional and unintentional injuries in a global community. Forensic nurses collaborate with agents in healthcare, social, and legal systems to investigate and interpret clinical presentations and pathologies by evaluating physical and psychological injury, whether intentional or unintentional; describing the scientific relationships of the injury and evidence; and interpreting the associated influencing factors.

Forensic nurses integrate forensic and nursing sciences in their assessment and care of victims and perpetrators of physical, psychological, or social trauma. Privacy, respect, and dignity characterize the services that forensic nursing provides to those affected by crime, trauma, and intentional harm. Forensic nurses are also strong advocates for minimum standards of assessment, evidence collection, and reporting of crime.

The current definition of forensic nursing adopted by the International Association of Forensic Nurses (2008) states: *Forensic nursing is the practice of nursing globally when health and legal systems intersect.*

Forensic Nursing Practice within Intersecting Systems

Forensic nurses provide care throughout the domains of nursing practice, education, research, and consultation (ANA & IAFN, 1997; IAFN, 2004). Furthermore, forensic nurses practice independently and collaboratively as needed in various settings whenever and wherever health and legal issues intersect. Forensic nurses interact with other systems in healthcare, community, and legal environments, including:

- Hospital and pre-hospital settings and clinics
- Legal or investigative arenas
- Commercial and not-for-profit enterprises, governments
- Educational, industrial, and correctional institutions

The systems in which forensic nurses practice vary depending on location, funding sources, community standards, and legal influences, and include:

- Healthcare (hospitals, surgery centers, community clinics)
- Investigative (medical examiner, law enforcement offices)
- Criminal justice (district attorney, public defender offices),
- Correctional (jails, prisons, and detention centers)
- Government (military, local, state, provincial, and federal agencies)

In addition, forensic nurse entrepreneurs establish businesses that focus on their forensic nursing practice and consultation expertise. Forensic nursing practice settings are evolving and increasing in number and variety.

The *core* of forensic nursing specifies the definitions, roles, behaviors, and processes inherent in forensic nursing practice. The *boundaries* of forensic nursing are both internal and external, with sufficient resilience to change in response to societal needs and demands. The *intersections* reflect overlap in boundaries for the forensic nurse with other professional groups by virtue of nursing's unique application of a common body of knowledge, environment, and focus. *Specialization* in forensic nursing incorporates a multitude of sub-specialty areas specific to the forensic health needs of patients in communities and across settings, populations, and systems.

Focus of Practice of Forensic Nurses

Forensic nurses are among the most diverse groups of clinicians in the nursing profession with respect to patient populations served, practice settings, and forensic and healthcare services provided. Yet all forensic nurses share skills and a body of knowledge related to the identification, assessment, and analysis of forensic patient data. They all apply a unique combination of processes rooted in nursing science, forensic science, and public health to care for patients.

Forensic nurses care for and treat individuals, families, communities, and populations in systems where intentional and unintentional injuries occur. These include but are not limited to patients who have been:

- Victims or perpetrators of interpersonal violence (e.g., child abuse, intimate partner abuse and assault, rape, gang violence, and government policy or legislation related to the violence),

- Victims or perpetrators of man-made catastrophe (e.g., automobile accidents, acts of terrorism), and

- Victims of natural causes of trauma and population evacuation (e.g., seismic or weather-related disasters).

Forensic nurses address the forensic healthcare needs of vulnerable and often disadvantaged patient populations (e.g., children, individuals with congenital and developmental handicaps, residents of nursing homes, psychiatric patients, and individuals who are addicted, homeless, or incarcerated). Forensic nurses also respond to community forensic and healthcare needs by concentrating on programmatic and systems change in the event of threats to public health and safety (e.g., reacting to environmental hazards with holistic death and mass-casualty incident investigations, forensic nursing programs and education, and policy and program development and legislation) where patients are affected by legal systems.

Patient populations cared for by forensic nurses are among the most vulnerable, disparaged, and disadvantaged in society. Forensic populations need social and legal systems to collaborate with health care to provide solutions for the identification and prevention of intentional and unintentional injury to individuals, families, communities, and social systems. Forensic nurses have both fundamental and specialized nursing knowledge and skills, including an understanding of the health-care, social, and legal systems that incorporates knowledge about forensic and public health science. Forensic nurses collaborate with agents in health, social, governmental, and legal systems to investigate and interpret clinical presentations and pathologies. Forensic nurses accomplish this by evaluating physical and psychological injury, whether intentional and unintentional, describing the scientific relationships of the injury and evidence, and interpreting the factors that influence them. Forensic nurses are experts across practice settings.

A key domain in forensic nursing practice is that of responding to the trauma of sexual assault and abuse and intervening through actions in systems to mitigate the impact of sexual violence on individuals, families, communities, and society. Forensic nurses provide care for victims of sexual assault in a variety of settings, including emergency departments or clinics (Ledray, 1999). The forensic nurse who has completed special education as a *sexual assault nurse examiner* (SANE) is an expert in history taking, assessment, treatment of trauma response and injury, documentation and collection of evidence and its management, emotional and social support required during a post-trauma evaluation and examination, and the documentation of injury and testimony required to bring such cases through the legal system (Speck & Peters, 1999). Unlike the nurse in the emergency room or clinic, the SANE is versed in the use of cutting-edge technology and techniques related to nursing assessment.

Another distinctive aspect of the SANE role is the use of a humane and legally objective approach that integrates advocacy and observation, evidentiary collection, mitigation of and protection against adverse health outcomes, including vicarious trauma, and location of community resources to support the victim. Accordingly, the SANE will have education and certification that reflects specialized knowledge about legal systems, evidence and ethical parameters, pathophysiology and injury and potential for injury, reproductive health, epidemiology, and technology and psychology associated with sexual assault, along with specialized training about the unique victim or offender population served.

The SANE role comes together most clearly in the medical assessment and treatment of the patient. While this is identical in terms of general nursing care, (e.g., assessment, planning, intervention, and evaluation), the SANE will also be responsible for representing the forensic nurse's encounter to the courts and society. This may include not only the evaluation and treatment of the patient's health status and bio-psycho-social-spiritual responses, but the health and forensic assessment, including history taking, evidence collection, and evidentiary outcomes. It will also include the systems response to the sexual assault in the courts and the community at large.

Evolution of Forensic Nursing

These key events in the development of forensic nursing highlight critical steps in the formalization of forensic nursing:

- In 1948, Article V in the Universal Declaration of Human Rights declared that "No one shall be subjected to torture or to cruel, inhuman or degrading treatment or punishment" (United Nations, 1948).
- In 1984 the U.S. Surgeon General identified violence as a public health issue, and healthcare providers as key agents in ameliorating the effects of violence in our communities (Koop, 1986).
- In 1991 AACN published a position paper stating that violence against women is a nursing practice issue (AACN, 1991).
- In 1991, Virginia Lynch's master's thesis conceptualized the "forensic nurse" (IAFN, 2008).
- In 1992 the International Association of Forensic Nurses was established as the first professional nursing organization for forensic nurses (IAFN, 2008).
- In 1995, ANA recognized forensic nursing as a specialty (IAFN, 2006).

These milestones led forensic nurses to recognize their important roles in identification, management, and prevention of intentional and unintentional injuries in a global community. In addition, forensic nursing has traditionally claimed a role in the assessment and care of perpetrators of crime, trauma, and intentional harm, particularly those whose mental or emotional disorder is related to the commission of crimes.

IAFN supports the forensic nurse in the development of international professional networks, the recognition of and expansion of the unique aspects of forensic nursing practice, establishment of scope and standards of forensic nursing practice, and creation of credentialing processes for forensic nurses. In addition, forensic nurses assist in the creation and dissemination of new and existing evidence-based knowledge of interest to forensic nurses, encourage collaboration among nurses and specialty practices, and promote interprofessional collaboration.

For example, the roles of registered nurses providing basic or advanced nursing health care to populations of clients in correctional settings are primarily determined by the settings in which they practice and the healthcare needs of their patients. Specialized knowledge for correctional nurses includes policies and procedures aimed at meeting specific primary healthcare needs of their patients while satisfying the need for security and safety. The correctional nurse is responsible for promoting health, preventing illness, restoring health, and alleviating suffering of those in prisons, jails, and other forms of custody. The forensic nurse in a corrections setting, on the other hand, will have the knowledge and basic skills of the correctional nurse, but will deliver care through competencies defined by advanced knowledge of clinical pathology related to criminality, incorporation of specific assessment tools to plan care for individuals and populations, and knowledge of injury assessment and prevention for correctional populations (Mason & Mercer, 1996; Shives, 2008).

Whatever the practice setting, the forensic nurse integrates knowledge of criminal justice, victimization, and impact of secure environments in the planning and implementation of systems to manage injury, manipulation, victimization, and trauma in correctional settings. The forensic nurse implements evidence-based practice through specialized knowledge in the detection of malingering, identification of different etiologies of self-mutilation and other forms of self harm, and negotiation of space and logistics in the management of violence and group behavior in secure settings. Specialized knowledge of the risk of boundary violations among staff and patients, along with the identification and management of such incidents, is another area of forensic nursing in correctional settings.

Practice Characteristics and Skills of Forensic Nurses

Forensic nurses provide direct services to individuals, families, communities, and populations; they affect the systems in which they function.

In addition, forensic nurses provide consultative services to nursing, medical, social, and other healthcare and legal agencies and the professionals in those agencies. The forensic nurse also provides factual and expert court testimony in areas dealing with both intentional and unintentional injury of the living or deceased.

Forensic nurses involved in death investigation bring nursing skills of observation, data collection, and analysis to the determination of manner and cause of death. The object of the forensic nurse in this setting is to advocate for the patient (the deceased) through the application of nursing skills and knowledge. While many professionals are involved in death investigation, the forensic nurse who is also a death investigator brings to any consideration of the deceased a holistic bio-psycho-social-spiritual approach, which can include the relationships the nurse ihas been able to establish with surviving family and others during investigations. Forensic nurses have an obligation to consider health promotion beyond the present investigation using the outcomes of death. The forensic nurse investigating death promotes health among colleagues, families, and communities of the deceased through the manner and tone of investigation. The forensic nursing role includes preservation of dignity, caring, and protection of rights even after death.

The forensic nurse develops and evaluates programs of care related to intentional and unintentional injury, crime, victimization, violence, abuse, and exploitation at the individual, community, state, province, district, regional, national, and international levels.

For example, the registered nurse practicing in a risk management department in hospital settings develops protocols for the collection of data and responses to indicators of patient or staff risk in healthcare settings, including injuries and other issues related to patient safety. In contrast, the forensic nurse working in a healthcare setting investigates using forensic nursing expertise (e.g., knowledge of investigation, evidence, intentional and unintentional injury) in the investigation of injury and trauma and criminality as these items relate to specific populations, such as the elderly and disabled (Sheridan, 2004) or the unexpected deceased.

While the forensic nurse and the risk management nurse collaborate across legal, social, and healthcare systems to provide evidence-based data that support solutions to risk, the forensic nurse has special expertise in cases relevant to a legal tort, such as but not limited to murder, rape, or abuse. The forensic nurse has specialized education in the identification of indicators of criminal activity and risk for injury, and the ability to distinguish intentional from unintentional trauma or injury, not available to the risk management nurse. While a risk management nurse would focus on the epidemiological trail of a virus or bacterium in an open system, the forensic nurse would focus on the evidence of intentional harm by individuals or groups that contribute to infection spread or epidemic, i.e., terrorist contamination. These nurses may work in collaboration, or the forensic nurse may be the designated investigator in the healthcare system when intentional harm is suspected; additionally, the forensic nurse can serve in a consultant role to the institution when intentional harm is suspected (e.g., unexpected death). The forensic nurse would also make recommendations to mitigate the opportunity for intentional harm in systems that will implement recommended changes as a response to risk.

Another example is the psychiatric nurse who applies knowledge of psychiatric principles and nursing theory to the care of persons with psychological or mental disorder in acute care and community-based settings (Shives, 2008). The psychiatric nurse may encounter patients who, by virtue of their emotional or mental disorder, commit or are likely to commit crimes or trauma against another or themselves. The forensic nurse in psychiatric settings has specialized knowledge and competencies in the assessment, care, and evaluation of individuals with mental disorders as they relate to criminal behavior. The forensic nurse will apply principles of forensic psychiatry and nursing to the clinical evaluation for competency and in the assessment and treatment of individuals and groups with crime-related mental disorders. The forensic nurse is a specialist in the care of the mentally disordered in secure settings, refining the care of such cases as self-injurious behavior and increased risk of victimization in secure settings (Mason & Mercer, 1996). The forensic nurse implements specialized instrumentation for the prediction of violence, assessment of self-harm risk, and determination of competency. The forensic nurse in this role has formal graduate nursing education with emphasis on forensic nursing care and interpersonal skills in systems responding to psychological trauma and abuse, neuropathology and criminology, and role transitions in victims and aggressors, where forensic nursing skills are practiced in secure settings and with the criminally mentally disordered.

Individual forensic nursing practice clearly differs according to both the nurse's experience and educational preparation and the characteristics of the patient population being served. Other major factors include the cultural, social, and legal systems in the forensic nursing practice setting.

This section has described the extensive range of forensic nursing practice. The following list conveys a similarly significant diversity of skills of the forensic nurse:

- Application of public health and forensic principles to the registered nursing practice, including bio-psycho-social-spiritual aspects of forensic nursing care in the scientific investigation/evaluation, diagnosis, treatment, and prevention of trauma and/or death of victims and perpetrators, including the measurement of outcomes and outputs of the practice.

- Development and implementation of systems relevant to forensic nursing, including development of systems that care for individuals, families, and communities as it relates to injury, both intentional and unintentional, to the care of individuals, families, communities or populations involved with criminal justice systems, and to measure the quality and safety outcomes.

- Development of quality forensic nursing care strategies through evidence-based practice and inquiry that target prevention of injury, both intentional and unintentional.

- Development, analysis, and implementation of health policy relevant to forensic nurses and forensic populations in forensic settings.

- Development and implementation of ethically sound, evidence-based, and culturally relevant processes within forensic nursing settings and systems.

- Development, analysis, reporting, and dissemination of relevant forensic data, evidence-based outcomes, and outputs.

- Identification, collection, and organization of data relevant to forensic nurses.

- Provision of testimony, both fact and expert, in judicial settings, competency hearings, and other venues.

- Design, evaluation, reporting, implementation, and dissemination of evidence-based and peer-reviewed research relevant to forensic nurses.

- Analysis of outcomes and influence in justice systems and on legislation that pertains to forensic nursing practice and healthcare quality, safety, outcomes, and outputs.

- Consultation with nursing practice communities and the interprofessional communities of medicine, legal systems, governments, and their agents.

- Interprofessional collaboration with justice, political and social systems, and the individuals who work in those systems.

- Quality education of various disciplines regarding forensic nursing practice.

- Leadership, administration, and management within forensic and healthcare settings.

- Evidence-based investigative and forensic interviewing.

- Forensic medical interviews for the purpose of diagnosis, treatment, and/or referral.

- Evaluation of crime scenes and trauma within settings relevant to the forensic nurse.

- Analysis of forensic healthcare quality through continuous review processes.

- Provision of evidence-based and safe direct patient care related to injury, crime, victimization, violence, abuse, and exploitation.

- Provision of evidence-based and safe forensic mental health care.

- Collection and preservation of forensic evidence.

- Integration of evidence-based forensic nursing practice to improve care of the forensic patient.

- Creation and implementation in forensic nursing systems and environments to improve the quality of forensic patient care, safety, and outcomes.

Educational Preparation and Credentialing of the Forensic Nurse

Historically, registered nurses have refined and developed their forensic nursing skills through clinical practice and continuing education. Today, there are five primary routes for preparation in forensic nursing (Burgess, Berger, & Boersma, 2004):

1. *Continuing education coursework* - Nurses can gain additional skills and knowledge about topics of interest to forensic nurses through continuing education courses (CEU).

2. *Certificate programs* - These include content relevant to the forensic nurse, set entrance requirements, and often provide clinical internships that result in a certificate detailing the completion of course work.

3. *Undergraduate nursing education* - Undergraduate academic programs in accredited schools of nursing offer electives, minors, or concentrations in forensic nursing that can contribute to a degree in nursing.

4. *Graduate nursing education* - The knowledge and skills acquired in baccalaureate and pre-licensure nursing programs are enhanced in formal graduate study. Following matriculation and completion of the forensic core content and prescribed forensic clinical experiences, the forensic nurse receives a master's or doctoral degree in the specialty of nursing.

5. *Post-doctoral education or fellowships* - The specific content and skills acquired in the terminal nursing degree programs are enhanced by formal forensic nursing core content and prescribed forensic clinical experiences. The programs may award diplomas.

Universities, schools of nursing, community colleges, and continuing education providers offer formal education opportunities for the specialty called forensic nursing at all academic levels. Entry-level schools of nursing offer introductory classes as electives. Accredited academic institutions offer degrees and certificates at graduate levels. Some forensic nursing education is provided by state and local government agencies, as well as by entrepreneurs. IAFN has published core domains, content, and performance measures in an outline of the curriculum for nursing educators and forensic nurses in practice (2004).

The forensic nurse brings all of the expertise of the professional nurse to the practice of forensic nursing. Entry-level practice requires completion of a basic nursing program leading to licensure as a registered nurse. Forensic nursing education focuses on injury and outcomes unique to forensic patients involved with the legal system either as victims or perpetrators or both. These areas include unique forensic terminology; intentional and unintentional injury; prevention; identification, diagnosis, treatment, and management of patients who include individuals, families, communities, and systems; psychology and psychopathology; and victimology. The principles of forensic nursing education are rooted in nursing and borrowed from public health and forensic science (Speck, 2000). Forensic nursing practice is summarized in the concepts of Wounding and Healing, Ethics, and Evidence, coupled with a fundamental understanding of the law and Legal processes (WHEEL); these principles are essential to the comprehensive practice of forensic nursing (Speck, 2000).

A forensic nurse has a lifelong commitment to learning which is necessary to remain current in clinical practice and legal issues that bear on the practice of the forensic nurse. Continuing education is required by many state or provincial governments to maintain licensure and certification. Education that is current and reflects evidence-based practice is necessary to ensure safe healthcare delivery and advocacy for patients and employers. Annual conferences, special forensic nursing interest group meetings, and educational programs and scientific publications serve as educational resources for practitioners at all levels of education, and document experience in the forensic nursing specialty. Issues such as differences in judicial processes among local, state, provincial, regional, national, and international venues; dissemination of advances in forensic science and forensic nursing science; and the evolutionary revisions to healthcare standards pose educational challenges to the forensic nurse of the future.

Forensic nurses demonstrate competency to the public through recognition and pursuit of excellence in practice. Credentialing, such as portfolio-building or certification in forensic nursing, is considered a priority for the specialty and is based on the identification of practice competencies and skills reflective of evidence-based practice. The forensic nurse demonstrates expertise in a forensic nursing role through credentialing designed to recognize clinical experience, knowledge, and heuristic practice wisdom. The forensic nurse acquires and maintains the credentials made available through certifying bodies of the forensic specialty and contributes to the evidence-based knowledge, standards, and criteria for specialty certification.

Certification offers tangible recognition of professional achievement in a defined functional or clinical area of nursing, such as forensic nursing. Through processes like portfolio-building or through examination for certification, forensic nurses earn credentials that are recognized within the profession and to consumers of the professional forensic nursing practice. The portfolio process for credentialing includes education, clinical hours of practice, peer evaluation of clinical competency, and demonstration of theoretical knowledge.

Levels of Forensic Nursing Practice

There are two levels of practice: basic and advanced.

Basic Forensic Nursing Practice

Basic forensic nursing is practiced by registered nurses who have knowledge and skills necessary for a specific role in forensic nursing, such as sexual assault nurse examiner (SANE). Basic forensic nursing practice is considered generalist and is guided by forensic nursing protocols for specific forensic populations of patients. Basic forensic nurses achieve specialized competencies through training programs, continuing education, and certification programs. Most generalists practicing basic forensic nursing are prepared for their nursing career at the diploma, associate degree, and bachelor's degree level.

For instance, a generalist forensic nurse specializing as a SANE will be licensed as an RN. After completing a SANE program and supervised patient encounters, the nurse will be eligible to sit for a certifying examination offered by the IAFN Forensic Nursing Certification Board. The certified SANE will receive victims of sexual assault and practice in a setting, such as emergency rooms, that is commensurate with nursing education and experience, within the scope of practice defined by professional organizations, regulatory agencies, and their institution.

Advanced Practice Forensic Nursing

Advanced practice forensic nursing incorporates expanded and specialized knowledge and skills. It is characterized by the integration and application of a range of theoretical and evidence-based knowledge acquired as a part of an advanced practice nursing graduate education. Forensic Advanced Practice Registered Nurses hold master's or doctorate degrees and are licensed, certified, and approved to practice in their roles as a clinical nurse specialist, nurse practitioner, or certified nurse midwife.

The advanced practice registered nurse or the Forensic Advanced Nursing Practice Nurse prepared as a SANE would hold a graduate degree at a minimum, or teach in a graduate curriculum in nursing with formal coursework in forensic sciences and public health or related theory, and forensic nursing applications. The graduate forensic nurse will be able to meet competencies identified in *Forensic Nursing: Scope and Standards of Practice* as well as domains located in the Core Curriculum for Forensic Advanced Practice Registered Nurses (IAFN, 2004). The practice of the forensic nurse who has a graduate nursing degree and is a SANE will differ from the generalist practice in the depth and breadth of knowledge on which nursing practice is based, and the scope of the role expectations. The graduate- or doctorate-prepared SANE would develop, promote, and implement evidence-based practice for individuals and families within systems. In addition, the graduate- or doctorate-prepared SANE would engage in research and formative and summative program evaluation in systems of care for victims and perpetrators of sexual assault and the complex health problems associated with sexual assault for individuals, families, and communities. Health promotion activities provided by the graduate- or doctorate-prepared SANE emphasize the identification and prevention of sexual assault and the resulting trauma and injury, as well as influencing systems change necessary to respond to this complex patient phenomenon in all types of communities.

In other cases, the Forensic Advanced Practice Registered Nurse collaborates with criminal justice and healthcare professionals to care for, diagnose, and treat patients impacted by injury, including follow-up care. The Forensic Advanced Practice Registered Nurse must obtain a minimum of a graduate degree in nursing with emphasis in an acknowledged specialty area (e.g., family nurse practitioner) on the prevention of trauma and the diagnosis and treatment of illnesses and responses to trauma, violence, and injury. The Forensic Advanced Practice Registered Nurse diagnoses, treats, and manages acute illness and chronic responses to injury in individuals, groups, and communities in the context of the medico-legal system. The assessment process would include obtaining health and forensic histories and conducting health and medical assessments for diagnostic purposes that include evidence collection and treatment of health outcomes. The Forensic Advanced Practice Registered Nurse prescribes medications and develops healthcare interventions within the scope of practice defined by professional organizations, regulatory agencies, and institutions. Health promotion activities of the advanced practice registered nurse and the Forensic Advanced Nursing Practice Nurse emphasize the identification and prevention of risks associated with violence, trauma, and injury in systems that respond to care of patients.

Ethics and Forensic Nursing

Based on the belief that human worth is the philosophical foundation on which forensic nursing is based, the practice of forensic nursing is consistent with IAFN's *Code of Ethics for Forensic Nurses* (2006), the *International Code of Ethics for Nurses* (ICNurses, 2006), and the *Code of Ethics for Nurses with Interpretative Statements* (ANA, 2001, 2005a)

Forensic nurses demonstrate an awareness of and adherence to regional and international laws governing their practice. Forensic nurses uphold ethical principles promoted by the nursing profession that protect the rights of, and advocate for, individuals, families, and communities in the systems that respond to them. The forensic nurse seeks evidence-based resources related to the health, safety, legal, and ethical issues for the forensic patient. Forensic nurses deliver services in a non-judgmental and non-discriminatory manner that is sensitive to diversity of the patient and the community. The forensic nurse practices with compassion and respect for the uniqueness of patients, including the moral and legal rights associated with self-determination within forensic settings and systems. Forensic nurses collaborate to address the forensic health needs of the patient, but when conflicting situations arise from previous bias and victimization, addiction, vicarious trauma, or interprofessional situations, the forensic nurse will examine the conflicts between personal and professional values, strive to preserve the patient's best interest, and preserve their professional integrity by establishing boundaries.

Nurses have a lifelong commitment to learning and maintenance of competence. This includes self-evaluation, coupled with peer review, to ensure that the forensic nursing practice is held to the highest standard. Nurses are required to have knowledge relevant to the current forensic nursing scope and standards of practice, including relevant changing issues, forensic nursing and nursing ethics, concerns, and controversies. Forensic nurses participate in the advancement of practice through administration, education, and knowledge development as well as advancing the profession through healthcare policy, professional standards, and dissemination of knowledge germane to forensic nursing practice. This may come from shared domains in nursing (such as public health, genetics and genomics) or other professions (such as medicine, public health, and forensic science). Most importantly, the forensic nurse has responsibilities to the public to respond appropriately to improve access to forensic nursing care and to bring about social change that creates a world without violence (ANA, 2001, 2005a; Canadian Nurses Association, 2002; IAFN, 2006; ICN, 2006).

Goals, Trends, and Issues in Forensic Nursing

The needs and expectations of society will shape the future of the specialty in a technologically savvy environment. Collaborating individuals, communities, organizations, and governments who support the development of the forensic nursing role will bring the forensic nurse specialist international recognition. The specialty knowledge, with acceptance and understanding of the scope and standards of practice, will continue to improve the response to patients who need forensic healthcare in interprofessional systems worldwide.

Education

Forensic nursing educational programs will continue to grow as an increasing number of accredited universities and colleges develop master's and doctorate curricula in the specialty of forensic nursing worldwide (AACN, 1998, 2006). The master's and doctorate education will reflect the expansion of the scientific evidence base of forensic nursing. Forensic nursing education will follow the trends for specialties using distance learning based on advanced technology, electronically supported simulations, and telemedicine. This trend will support access to education for and by master's and doctorate forensic nurses in remote locations worldwide and, in turn, will provide access to quality forensic nursing care to the patient populations residing in their remote communities. Future forensic nurses will assume leadership positions and create new venues for forensic nurse practice, such as entrepreneurial activities and legislative representation. Future forensic nurses will influence nursing practice because at all levels of nursing education, elements of forensic nursing content are and will continue to be threaded throughout nursing coursework.

Research

Research, as a foundation for evidence-based practice, supports the forensic nurse role. With technological advances in informatics and communication, forensic nursing research will develop at a rapid pace as clinical, educational, and administrative Forensic Advanced Practice Registered Nurses will require and produce scientific evidence in support of their growing practices. Informatics will provide the conduit for the rapid dissemination of forensic nursing research (O'Carroll & Public Health Informatics Competencies Working Group, 2002). Forensic nursing research will influence government policy, legislation, and action as the scientific base increases and graduate education, experience, and credentialing processes are realized by the forensic nursing community. It is also projected that the international interprofessional community will increasingly acknowledge the forensic nurse as a valuable interprofessional team member where healthcare and legal systems intersect.

Population Focus

Forensic nursing and public health nursing are inextricably linked both locally and in international cultures and systems, particularly in the primary, secondary, and tertiary care of intentional and unintentional injury involving individuals, families, communities, and populations. Future master's and doctorate curriculums internationally will use the graduate public health nursing competencies (QUAD Council, 2003) as a basis for forensic care of populations by nurses, an essential requirement in master's and doctorate education competencies (AACN, 2006). In addition, the population emphasis on prevention, health promotion, and program formative and summative evaluation and sustainability will help meet pressing needs in patient populations at risk for injury from intentional and unintentional violence. The population-focused approaches toward man-made or weather-related disaster and mass casualty will merge population care with intentional and unintentional injury aspects of the two disciplines—forensic nursing and public health nursing. The forensic nursing specialist will influence policy, practice, and trends when tackling issues of population-focused care related to intentional and unintentional injury prevention and intervention. As a well-educated and respected professional, the graduate forensic nurse will link public health principles and forensic science to forensic nursing practice to create a foundation for the evaluation and treatment of injury in populations worldwide.

Genetics and Genomics

Technology will provide future forensic nurses with tremendous information about patients affected by genetic healthcare problems who seek care in a forensic setting (Consensus Panel, 2006). With the integration of genetic and genomic knowledge in nursing curricula, future forensic nurses will understand the relationships between health and genetics and genomics as it relates to violence, violent behavior, and victimization. Forensic nurses will also provide services based on culture, religion, knowledge level, literacy, and preferred language in the context of the forensic healthcare presentation in the patient, whether individual, family, community, or population.

STANDARDS OF FORENSIC NURSING PRACTICE

Function of Standards

The Standards, which are comprised of the standards of practice (pages 23–34) and the standards of professional performance (pages 35–48), are authoritative statements by which nurses practicing within the role, population, and specialty governed by this document (*Forensic Nursing: Scope and Standards of Practice*) that describe the duties that they are expected to competently perform. The Standards published herein may be utilized as evidence of the legal standard of care governing nurses practicing within the role, population, and specialty governed by this document. The Standards are subject to change with the dynamics of the nursing profession and as new patterns of professional practice are developed and accepted by the nursing profession and the public. In addition, specific conditions and clinical circumstances may also affect the application of the Standards at a given time; e.g., during a natural disaster. The Standards are subject to formal, periodic review and revision.

The measurement criteria that appear below each standard are not all-inclusive and do not establish the legal standard of care. Rather, the measurement criteria are specific, measurable elements that can be used by nursing professionals to measure professional performance. Nurses practicing within this particular role, population, and specialty can identify opportunities for development and improvement by evaluating performance on these elements.

Appendix B. Forensic Nursing: Scope and Standards of Practice (2009)

STANDARDS OF PRACTICE

STANDARD 1. ASSESSMENT
The forensic nurse collects comprehensive data pertinent to the patient's health or the situation.

Measurement Criteria:

The forensic nurse:

- Collects data in a systematic and ongoing process with a focus on identifying the medical–legal implications of those findings.

- Involves the patient, family, community, nurses and other healthcare providers, interprofessional personnel, and environment, as appropriate, in collaborative holistic data collection.

- Prioritizes data collection activities based on the patient's immediate condition, anticipated needs of the patient or situation, and preservation of legal evidence.

- Uses appropriate evidence-based assessment techniques and instruments in collecting pertinent data.

- Uses analytical models and problem-solving tools in forensic nursing practice.

- Synthesizes available data, information, and knowledge relevant to the situation to identify patterns and variances.

- Documents relevant data in a retrievable format.

Additional Measurement Criteria for the Forensic Advanced Practice Registered Nurse:

The Forensic Advanced Practice Registered Nurse:

- Initiates and interprets diagnostic tests and procedures relevant to the specific area of forensic nursing practice.

Standard 2. Diagnosis

The forensic nurse analyzes the assessment data to determine the diagnoses or issues.

Measurement Criteria:

The forensic nurse:

- Derives the diagnoses or issues based on assessment data.

- Validates the diagnoses or issues with the patient, family, and other healthcare providers when possible and appropriate.

- Documents diagnoses or issues in a manner that facilitates the determination of the expected outcomes and plan.

Additional Measurement Criteria for the Forensic Advanced Practice Registered Nurse:

The Forensic Advanced Practice Registered Nurse:

- Systematically compares and contrasts clinical findings with normal and abnormal variations and developmental events in formulating a differential diagnosis.

- Utilizes complex data and information obtained during interview, examination, diagnostic procedures, and review of medical–legal evidentiary documents in identifying diagnoses.

- Assists staff in developing and maintaining competency in the diagnostic process.

STANDARD 3. OUTCOMES IDENTIFICATION

The forensic nurse identifies expected outcomes for a plan individualized to the patient or the situation.

Measurement Criteria:

The forensic nurse:

- Involves the patient, family, other healthcare providers, and other collaborating professionals, in formulating expected outcomes when possible and appropriate.

- Derives culturally appropriate expected outcomes from the diagnoses.

- Considers associated risks, benefits, costs, current scientific evidence, medical–legal factors, and clinical expertise when formulating expected outcomes.

- Defines expected outcomes in terms of the patient, patient values, ethical considerations, environment, or situation with such considerations as associated risks, benefits and costs, and current scientific evidence.

- Includes a time estimate for attainment of expected outcomes when appropriate.

- Develops expected outcomes that provide direction for continuity of care.

- Modifies expected outcomes based on changes in the status of the patient or evaluation of the situation.

- Documents expected outcomes as measurable goals.

Additional Measurement Criteria for the Forensic Advanced Practice Registered Nurse:

The Forensic Advanced Practice Registered Nurse:

- Identifies expected outcomes that incorporate scientific evidence and are achievable through implementation of evidence-based practices.

- Identifies expected outcomes that incorporate cost and clinical effectiveness, patient satisfaction, community safety, and continuity and consistency among providers.

- Supports the use of clinical guidelines linked to positive patient outcomes.

Standard 4. Planning

The forensic nurse develops a plan that prescribes strategies and alternatives to attain expected outcomes.

Measurement Criteria:

The forensic nurse:

- Develops an individualized plan considering patient characteristics or the situation (e.g., age- and culturally appropriate, environmentally sensitive).
- Develops the plan in conjunction with the patient, family, and others, as appropriate.
- Includes strategies in the plan that address each of the identified diagnoses or issues, which may include strategies for promotion and restoration of health and prevention of illness, injury, and disease.
- Provides for continuity in the plan.
- Incorporates an implementation pathway or timeline in the plan.
- Establishes the plan priorities with the patient, family, and others as appropriate.
- Utilizes the plan to provide direction to other members of the healthcare and interprofessional team.
- Defines the plan to reflect current statutes, rules and regulations, and standards.
- Integrates current trends and research affecting care in planning.
- Considers the economic impact of the plan.
- Uses standardized language or recognized terminology to document the plan.

Additional Measurement Criteria for the Forensic Advanced Practice Registered Nurse:

The Forensic Advanced Practice Registered Nurse:

- Identifies assessment and diagnostic strategies and therapeutic interventions in the plan that reflect current evidence, including data, research, literature, and expert clinical knowledge.

- Selects or designs strategies to meet the multifaceted needs of complex patients and situations.
- Includes the synthesis of patients' values and beliefs regarding nursing and medical therapies in the plan.

Additional Measurement Criteria for the Nursing Role Specialty:

The forensic nurse in a nursing role specialty:

- Participates in the design and development of interprofessional and multi/inter-disciplinary processes to address the forensic situation or issue.
- Contributes to the development, evaluation, and continuous improvement of organizational systems that support planning.
- Supports the integration of clinical, human, medical–legal, social, and financial resources to enhance and complete decision-making.

Standard 5. Implementation
The forensic nurse implements the identified plan.

Measurement Criteria:

The forensic nurse:

- Implements the plan in a safe and timely manner.
- Documents implementation and any modifications, including changes or omissions, of the identified plan.
- Utilizes evidence-based interventions and treatments specific to the diagnosis or problem.
- Utilizes community resources and systems to implement the plan.
- Collaborates with nursing colleagues and others to implement the plan.

Additional Measurement Criteria for the Forensic Advanced Practice Registered Nurse:

The Forensic Advanced Practice Registered Nurse:

- Facilitates modification and utilization of systems and community resources to implement the plan.
- Supports collaboration with nursing colleagues and other disciplines and professions to implement the plan.
- Incorporates new knowledge and strategies to initiate change in nursing care practices if desired outcomes are not achieved.

Additional Measurement Criteria for the Nursing Role Specialty:

The forensic nurse in a nursing role specialty:

- Implements the plan using principles and concepts of project or systems management.
- Fosters organizational systems that support implementation of the plan.

Standard 5a: Coordination of Care
The forensic nurse coordinates care delivery.

Measurement Criteria:

The forensic nurse:

- Coordinates implementation of the plan.
- Documents the coordination of the care and the plan.

Measurement Criteria for the Forensic Advanced Practice Registered Nurse:

The Forensic Advanced Practice Registered Nurse:

- Provides leadership in the administration and coordination of interprofessional health care for integrated delivery of patient care services.
- Synthesizes data and information to prescribe necessary system and community support measures, including environmental modifications.
- Coordinates system and community resources that enhance delivery of care across continuums.

STANDARD 5B: HEALTH TEACHING AND HEALTH PROMOTION

The forensic nurse employs strategies to promote health and a safe environment.

Measurement Criteria:

The forensic nurse:

- Provides health teaching that addresses such topics as healthy lifestyles, risk-reducing behaviors, developmental needs, activities of daily living, and preventive self care.

- Uses health promotion and health teaching methods appropriate to the situation and the patient's developmental level, learning needs, readiness, ability to learn, language preference, and culture.

- Seeks opportunities for feedback and evaluation of the effectiveness of the strategies used.

Additional Measurement Criteria for the Forensic Advanced Practice Registered Nurse:

The Forensic Advanced Practice Registered Nurse:

- Synthesizes empirical evidence on risk behaviors, learning theories, behavioral change theories, motivational theories, epidemiology, and other related theories and frameworks when designing health information and patient education.

- Designs health information and patient education appropriate to the patient's developmental level, learning needs, readiness to learn, and cultural values and beliefs.

- Evaluates health information resources, such as the Internet, in the area of practice for accuracy, readability, and comprehensibility to help patients access quality health information.

Appendix B. Forensic Nursing: Scope and Standards of Practice (2009)

STANDARD 5C: CONSULTATION

The Forensic Advanced Practice Registered Nurse and the nursing role specialist provide consultation to influence the identified plan, enhance the abilities of others, and effect change.

Measurement Criteria for the Forensic Advanced Practice Registered Nurse:

The Forensic Advanced Practice Registered Nurse:

- Synthesizes clinical data, theoretical frameworks, and evidence when providing consultation.

- Facilitates the effectiveness of a consultation by involving the patient in making decisions and negotiating role responsibilities.

- Communicates consultation recommendations that facilitate change.

Measurement Criteria for the Nursing Role Specialty

The forensic nurse in a nursing role specialty:

- Synthesizes data, information, theoretical frameworks, and evidence when providing consultation.

- Facilitates the effectiveness of a consultation by involving the stakeholders in the decision-making process.

- Communicates consultation recommendations that influence the identified plan, facilitate understanding by involved stakeholders, enhance the work of others, and effect change.

STANDARD 5D: PRESCRIPTIVE AUTHORITY AND TREATMENT
The Forensic Advanced Practice Registered Nurse uses prescriptive authority, procedures, referrals, treatments, and therapies in accordance with state and federal laws and regulations.

Measurement Criteria for the Forensic Advanced Practice Registered Nurse:
The Forensic Advanced Practice Registered Nurse:

- Prescribes evidence-based treatments, therapies, and procedures considering the patient's comprehensive healthcare needs.

- Prescribes pharmacologic agents based on a current knowledge of pharmacology and physiology.

- Prescribes specific pharmacological agents or treatments based on clinical indicators, the patient's status and needs, and the results of diagnostic and laboratory tests.

- Evaluates therapeutic and potential adverse effects of pharmacological and non-pharmacological treatments.

- Provides patients with information about intended effects and potential adverse effects of proposed prescriptive therapies.

- Provides information about costs and alternative treatments and procedures, as appropriate.

STANDARD **6.** EVALUATION

The forensic nurse evaluates progress towards attainment of outcomes.

Measurement Criteria:

The forensic nurse:

- Conducts a systematic, ongoing, and criterion-based evaluation of the outcomes in relation to the structures and processes prescribed by the plan and the indicated timeline.

- Includes the patient and others involved in the care or situation in the evaluation process.

- Evaluates the effectiveness of the planned strategies in relation to patient responses and the attainment of the expected outcomes.

- Documents the results of the evaluation.

- Uses ongoing assessment data to revise the diagnoses, outcomes, the plan, and the implementation as needed.

- Disseminates the results to the patient and others involved in the care or situation, as appropriate, in accordance with state and federal laws and regulations.

Additional Measurement Criteria for the Forensic Advanced Practice Registered Nurse:

The Forensic Advanced Practice Registered Nurse:

- Evaluates the accuracy of the diagnosis and the effectiveness of the interventions in relation to the patient's attainment of expected outcomes.

- Synthesizes the results of the evaluation analyses to determine the impact of the plan on the affected patients, families, groups, communities, and institutions.

- Uses the results of the evaluation analyses to make or recommend process or structural changes including policy, procedure, or protocol documentation, as appropriate.

Continued ▶

Additional Measurement Criteria for the Nursing Role Specialty:

The forensic nurse in a nursing role specialty:

- Uses the results of the evaluation analyses to make or recommend process or structural changes including policy, procedure, or protocol documentation, as appropriate.

- Synthesizes the results of the evaluation analyses to determine the impact of the plan on the affected patients, families, groups, communities, institutions, networks, and organizations.

STANDARDS OF PROFESSIONAL PERFORMANCE

STANDARD 7. QUALITY OF PRACTICE
The forensic nurse systematically enhances the quality and effectiveness of forensic nursing practice.

Measurement Criteria:

The forensic nurse:

- Demonstrates quality by documenting the application of the nursing process in a responsible, accountable, and ethical manner.

- Uses the results of quality improvement activities to initiate changes in forensic nursing practice and in the healthcare delivery system.

- Uses creativity and innovation in forensic nursing practice to improve care delivery.

- Incorporates new knowledge to initiate changes in forensic nursing practice if desired outcomes are not achieved.

- Participates in quality improvement activities such as:

  - Identifying aspects of forensic nursing practice important for quality monitoring.

  - Using indicators developed to monitor quality and effectiveness of forensic nursing practice.

  - Collecting data to monitor quality and effectiveness of forensic nursing practice.

  - Analyzing quality data to identify opportunities for improving forensic nursing practice.

  - Formulating recommendations to improve forensic nursing practice or outcomes.

  - Taking action to enhance the quality of forensic nursing practice.

  - Developing, implementing, and evaluating policies, procedures, and guidelines to improve the quality of forensic nursing practice.

Continued ▶

- Participating on interprofessional teams to evaluate clinical care or health services.
- Participating in efforts to minimize costs and unnecessary duplication.
- Analyzing factors related to safety, satisfaction, effectiveness, and cost–benefit options.
- Analyzing organizational systems for barriers.
- Implementing processes to remove or decrease barriers in organizational systems.

Additional Measurement Criteria for the Forensic Advanced Practice Registered Nurse:

The Forensic Advanced Practice Registered Nurse:

- Obtains and maintains professional certification if available in the area of expertise.
- Designs quality improvement initiatives.
- Implements initiatives to evaluate the need for change.
- Evaluates the practice environment and quality of nursing care rendered in relation to existing evidence, identifying opportunities for the generation and use of research.

Additional Measurement Criteria for the Nursing Role Specialty:

The forensic nurse in a nursing role specialty:

- Obtains and maintains professional certification if available in the area of expertise.
- Designs quality improvement initiatives.
- Implements initiatives to evaluate the need for change.
- Evaluates the practice environment in relation to existing evidence, identifying opportunities for the generation and use of research.

STANDARD 8. EDUCATION

The forensic nurse attains knowledge and competency that reflect current nursing practice.

Measurement Criteria:

The forensic nurse:

- Participates in ongoing educational activities related to appropriate knowledge bases and professional issues.
- Demonstrates a commitment to lifelong learning through self-reflection and inquiry to identify learning needs.
- Seeks experiences that reflect current practice in order to maintain skills and competence in clinical practice or role performance.
- Acquires knowledge and skills appropriate to the specialty area, practice setting, role, or situation.
- Maintains professional records that provide evidence of competency and lifelong learning.
- Seeks experiences and formal and independent learning activities to maintain and develop clinical and professional skills and knowledge.

Additional Measurement Criteria for the Forensic Advanced Practice Registered Nurse:

The Forensic Advanced Practice Registered Nurse:

- Uses current healthcare research findings and other evidence to expand clinical knowledge, enhance role performance, and increase knowledge of professional issues.

Additional Measurement Criteria for the Nursing Role Specialty:

The forensic nurse in a nursing role specialty:

- Uses current research findings and other evidence to expand knowledge, enhance role performance, and increase knowledge of professional issues.

STANDARD 9. PROFESSIONAL PRACTICE EVALUATION

The forensic nurse evaluates one's own nursing practice in relation to professional practice standards and guidelines, relevant statutes, rules, and regulations.

Measurement Criteria:

The forensic nurse's practice reflects the application of knowledge of current practice standards, guidelines, statutes, rules, and regulations. The forensic nurse:

- Provides age-appropriate care in a culturally and ethnically sensitive manner.

- Engages in self-evaluation of practice on a regular basis, identifying areas of strength as well as areas in which professional development would be beneficial.

- Obtains informal feedback regarding one's own practice from patients, peers, professional colleagues, and others.

- Participates in systematic peer review as appropriate.

- Takes action to achieve goals identified during the evaluation process.

- Provides rationales for practice beliefs, decisions, and actions as part of the informal and formal evaluation processes.

Additional Measurement Criteria for the Forensic Advanced Practice Registered Nurse:

The Forensic Advanced Practice Registered Nurse:

- Engages in a formal process seeking feedback regarding one's own practice from patients, peers, professional colleagues, and others.

Additional Measurement Criteria for the Nursing Role Specialty:

The forensic nurse in a nursing role specialty:

- Engages in a formal process seeking feedback regarding role performance from individuals, professional colleagues, representatives and administrators of corporate entities, and others.

STANDARD 10. COLLEGIALITY

The forensic nurse interacts with, and contributes to the professional development of, peers and colleagues.

Measurement Criteria:

The forensic nurse:

- Shares knowledge and skills with peers and colleagues as evidenced by such activities as patient care conferences or presentations at formal or informal meetings.
- Provides peers with feedback regarding their practice or role performance.
- Interacts with peers and colleagues to enhance one's own professional nursing practice and role performance.
- Maintains compassionate and caring relationships with peers and colleagues.
- Contributes to an environment that is conducive to the education of healthcare professionals.
- Contributes to a supportive and healthy work environment.

Additional Measurement Criteria for the Forensic Advanced Practice Registered Nurse:

The Forensic Advanced Practice Registered Nurse:

- Models expert practice to other nurses, interprofessional team members, and healthcare consumers.
- Mentors other registered nurses and colleagues as appropriate.
- Participates with teams that contribute to role development and advanced nursing practice and health care.

Additional Measurement Criteria for the Nursing Role Specialty:

The forensic nurse in a nursing role specialty:

- Participates on interprofessional and nursing teams that contribute to role development and, directly or indirectly, advance nursing practice and health services.
- Mentors other registered nurses and colleagues as appropriate.

Standard 11. Collaboration

The forensic nurse collaborates with patient, family, and others in the conduct of nursing practice.

Measurement Criteria:

The forensic nurse:

- Communicates with patient, family, and healthcare providers regarding patient care and the nurse's role in the provision of that care.

- Collaborates in creating a documented plan focused on outcomes and decisions related to care and delivery of services that indicates communication with patients, families, and others.

- Partners with others to effect change and generate positive outcomes through knowledge of the patient or situation.

- Documents referrals, including provisions for continuity of care.

Additional Measurement Criteria for the Forensic Advanced Practice Registered Nurse:

The Forensic Advanced Practice Registered Nurse:

- Partners with other disciplines to enhance patient care through interprofessional activities, such as education, consultation, management, technological development, or research opportunities.

- Facilitates an interprofessional process with other members of the healthcare team.

- Documents plan-of-care communications, rationales for plan-of-care changes, and collaborative discussions to improve patient care.

Additional Measurement Criteria for Nursing Role Specialty:

The forensic nurse in a nursing role specialty:

- Partners with others to enhance health care, and ultimately patient care, through interprofessional activities such as education, consultation, management, technological development, or research opportunities.

- Documents plans, communications, rationales for plan changes, and collaborative discussions.

STANDARD **12.** ETHICS

The forensic nurse integrates ethical provisions in all areas of practice.

Measurement Criteria:

The forensic nurse:

- Uses *Code of Ethics for Nurses with Interpretive Statements* (ANA, 2001) and *Forensic Nurse's Code of Ethics* (IAFN, 2006) to guide practice.
- Delivers care in a manner that protects patient autonomy, dignity, and rights.
- Maintains patient confidentiality within legal and regulatory parameters.
- Serves as a patient advocate assisting patients in developing skills for self-advocacy and empowerment.
- Maintains a therapeutic and professional patient–nurse relationship within appropriate professional role boundaries.
- Demonstrates a commitment to practicing self-care, managing stress, and connecting with self and others.
- Contributes to resolving ethical issues of patients, colleagues, or systems as evidenced in such activities as participating on ethics committees.
- Reports illegal, incompetent, or impaired practices.

Additional Measurement Criteria for the Forensic Advanced Practice Registered Nurse:

The Forensic Advanced Practice Registered Nurse:

- Informs the patient of the risks, benefits, and outcomes of health-care regimens.
- Participates in interprofessional and nursing teams that address ethical risks, benefits, and outcomes for patients.

Continued ▶

Additional Measurement Criteria for the Nursing Role Specialty:

The forensic nurse in a nursing role specialty:

- Participates on interprofessional teams that address ethical risks, benefits, and outcomes.
- Informs administrators or others of the risks, benefits, and outcomes of programs and decisions that affect healthcare delivery.

STANDARD 13. RESEARCH
The forensic nurse integrates research findings into practice.

Measurement Criteria:

The forensic nurse:

- Utilizes the best available evidence, including research findings, to guide practice decisions.

- Actively participates in research activities at various levels appropriate to the nurse's level of education and position. Such activities may include:

  - Identifying clinical problems specific to nursing research (patient care and forensic nursing practice).

  - Participating in data collection (such as, but not limited to surveys, pilot projects, formal studies).

  - Participating in formal committees or programs.

  - Sharing research and findings with peers and others.

  - Conducting research.

  - Critically analyzing and interpreting research for application to practice.

  - Using research findings in the development of policies, procedures, and standards of practice in patient care.

  - Incorporating research as a basis for learning.

Additional Measurement Criteria for the Forensic Advanced Practice Registered Nurse:

The Forensic Advanced Practice Registered Nurse:

- Contributes to nursing knowledge by conducting or synthesizing research that discovers, examines, and evaluates knowledge, theories, criteria, and creative approaches to improve healthcare practice.

- Formally disseminates research findings through activities such as presentations, publications, consultation, and journal clubs.

Continued ▶

Additional Measurement Criteria for the Nursing Role Specialty:

The forensic nurse in a nursing role specialty:

- Contributes to nursing knowledge by conducting or synthesizing research that discovers, examines, and evaluates knowledge, theories, criteria, and creative approaches to improve health care.
- Formally disseminates research findings through activities such as presentations, publications, consultation, and journal clubs.

STANDARD 14. RESOURCE UTILIZATION

The forensic nurse considers factors related to safety, effectiveness, cost, and impact on practice in the planning and delivery of nursing services.

Measurement Criteria:

The forensic nurse:

- Evaluates factors such as safety, effectiveness, availability, cost–benefits, efficiencies, and impact on practice, when choosing among practice options that would result in the same expected outcome.

- Assists the patient and family in identifying and securing appropriate and available services to address health-related needs.

- Assigns or delegates tasks, based on the needs and condition of the patient, potential for harm, stability of the patient's condition, complexity of the task, and predictability of the outcome.

- Assists the patient and family in becoming informed consumers about the options, costs, risks, and benefits of treatment and care.

Additional Measurement Criteria for the Forensic Advanced Practice Registered Nurse:

The Forensic Advanced Practice Registered Nurse:

- Utilizes organizational and community resources to formulate interprofessional plans of care.

- Develops innovative solutions for patient care problems that address effective resource utilization and maintenance of quality.

- Develops strategies to evaluate cost-effectiveness associated with nursing practice.

Additional Measurement Criteria for the Nursing Role Specialty:

The forensic nurse in a nursing role specialty:

- Develops innovative solutions and applies strategies to obtain appropriate resources for nursing initiatives.

Continued ▶

- Secures organizational resources to ensure a work environment conducive to completing the identified plan and outcomes.
- Develops formative and summative evaluation methods to measure safety and effectiveness for interventions and outcomes.
- Promotes activities that assist others, as appropriate, in becoming informed about costs, risks, and benefits of care or of the plan and solution.

STANDARD **15.** LEADERSHIP

The forensic nurse provides leadership in the professional practice setting and the profession.

Measurement Criteria:

The forensic nurse:

- Engages in teamwork as a team player and a team builder.
- Works to create and maintain healthy work environments in local, regional, national, or international communities.
- Displays the ability to define a clear vision, the associated goals, and a plan to implement and measure progress.
- Demonstrates a commitment to continuous, lifelong learning for self and others.
- Teaches others to succeed by mentoring and other strategies.
- Exhibits creativity and flexibility through times of change.
- Demonstrates energy, excitement, and a passion for quality work.
- Willingly accepts mistakes by self and others, thereby creating a culture in which risk-taking is not only safe, but expected.
- Inspires loyalty by valuing people as the most precious asset in an organization.
- Directs the coordination of care across settings and among caregivers, including oversight of licensed and unlicensed personnel in any assigned or delegated tasks.
- Serves in key roles in the work setting by assuming leadership positions on committees, councils, and administrative teams.
- Promotes advancement of the profession through active participation in professional organizations.

Continued ▶

Additional Measurement Criteria for the Forensic Advanced Practice Registered Nurse:

The Forensic Advanced Practice Registered Nurse:

- Works to influence decision-making bodies to improve patient care.
- Provides direction to enhance the effectiveness of the healthcare and interprofessional team.
- Initiates and revises protocols or guidelines to reflect evidence-based practice, to reflect accepted changes in care management, or to address emerging problems.
- Promotes communication of information and advancement of the profession through writing, publishing, and presentations for inter-professional or lay audiences.
- Designs innovations to effect change in practice and improves health outcomes.

Additional Measurement Criteria for the Nursing Role Specialty:

The forensic nurse in a nursing role specialty:

- Works to influence decision-making bodies to improve patient care, health services, and policies.
- Promotes communication of information and advancement of the profession through writing, publishing, and presentations for professional or lay audiences.
- Designs innovations to effect change in practice and outcomes.
- Provides evidence-based direction and leadership to enhance the effectiveness of interprofessional teams.

Glossary

Assessment. A systematic, dynamic process by which the registered nurse collects and analyzes data (ANA, 2004). In forensic settings: (1) the RN interacts with the patient, family, groups, communities, populations, healthcare providers, public health and law enforcement agencies, and medical and judicial systems; (2) may include these dimensions: physical, psychological, sociocultural, spiritual, cognitive, functional abilities, developmental, economic, cultural, and lifestyle.

Certification. Tangible recognition of professional achievement in a defined functional or clinical area of nursing (American Board of Nursing Specialties, 2005, n.d.).

Continuity of care. A process that involves patients, families, significant others, and interprofessional team members in the determination of a coordinated plan of care. This process facilitates the patient's transition between settings, healthcare providers, and interprofessional agencies, and is based on changing needs and available resources in the community.

Diagnosis. A judgment about the response to actual or potential health conditions or needs; the diagnosis provides the basis for determination of a plan of services to achieve expected outcomes; registered nurses in forensic settings utilize nursing or medical diagnoses depending on educational and clinical preparation and legal authority.

Environment. The atmosphere, milieu, or condition in which an individual lives, works, or plays (ANA, 2004).

Evaluation. The process of determining the progress toward the attainment of expected outcomes; outcomes include the effectiveness of care, when addressing one's practice (ANA, 2004).

Evidence-based practice. A process founded on the collection, interpretation, and integration of valid, important, and applicable patient-reported, clinician-observed, and research-derived evidence. The best available evidence, moderated by patient circumstances and preferences, is applied to improve the quality of clinical judgments (ANA, 2004).

Family. Family of origin or significant others as identified by the patient (ANA, 2004).

Forensic. Pertaining to law; for the purposes of this document, relating to the use of science or technology in the investigation and establishment of facts or evidence (Merriam-Webster's 2008).

Forensic Advanced Practice Registered Nurse. A licensed registered nurse who has completed graduate or doctoral education with a specialization or emphasis in forensic nursing, and holds Advanced Practice Registered Nurse (APRN) credentials as a Clinical Nurse Specialist, Certified Nurse-Midwife, or Nurse Practitioner.

Forensic nursing. "The practice of nursing globally where health and legal systems intersect" (IAFN, 2008).

Formative evaluation. The structured development of processes or programs including the goals, outcomes, and output identification (Weiss, 1998). In the forensic nursing process and programs this can inlcude setting program goals, objectives, developing measurement tools, and creating action plans that identify outcomes and outputs of the process or program.

Guidelines. Systematically developed statements that describe recommended actions based on available scientific evidence and expert opinion. Clinical guidelines describe a process of patient care management that has the potential of improving the quality of clinical and consumer decision making (ANA, 2004).

Holistic. Based on an understanding that the patient is an interconnected unity and that physical, mental, social, and spiritual factors need to be included in interventions (ANA, 2004).

Illness. The subjective experience of discomfort (ANA, 2004).

Implementation. Activities such as teaching, monitoring, providing, counseling, delegating, and coordinating (ANA, 2004) and , in forensic settings, administration.

Injury. Trauma; any damage or harm done to or suffered by a person or thing that involves the bio-psycho-social, spiritual, or financial state of an individual, family, community, or system for which legal redress may be available.

Appendix B. Forensic Nursing: Scope and Standards of Practice (2009)

Interprofessional. Founded on engagement between professions, such as prosecutors, law enforcement officers, nurses, judges, and police officers; or between physicians and nurses. (See also *Multidisciplinary*.)

Legal. Pertaining to the law; used for the purposes of this document as a broad term to describe criminal and civil justice systems and investigative disciplines.

Multidisciplinary. Reliance on each team member or discipline contributing discipline-specific skills (ANA, 2004); in forensic nursing, usually means *interprofessional*.

Nursing. Protection, promotion, and optimization of health and abilities, prevention of illness and injury, alleviation of suffering through the diagnosis and treatment of human response, and advocacy in the care of individuals, families, communities, and populations (ANA, 2003, 2004).

Offender. One who commits, executes, or performs a criminal act of any kind and whose profiles and treatment modalities are integral to forensic nursing practice. (See also *Perpetrator*.)

Outcomes. Measurable, expected goals.

Outputs. Measurable, tangible products.

Patient. The recipient of forensic nursing practice, whether an individual, family, community, or population. The recipient may also be called client, resident, group, or system (ANA, 2004).

- When the patient is an *individual*, the focus is the health state, problems, or needs of a single person.

- When the patient is a *family* or a *group*, the focus is on the health state of that unit as a whole or the reciprocal effects of any individual's health state on any other members of the unit.

- When the patient is a *community* or *population*, the focus is on personal and environmental health and the health risks of the community or entire population.

Peer review. A collegial, systematic, and periodic process by which registered nurses are held accountable for their practice and that fosters refinement of their knowledge, skills, and decision-making at all levels in all areas of work, such as in their nursing practice (ANA, 2004).

Perpetrator. One who commits, executes, or performs a criminal act of any kind and whose profiles and treatment modalities are integral to forensic nursing practice. (See also *Offender.*)

Plan. A comprehensive outline of the steps to be completed to attain expected outcomes (ANA, 2004). May include any or all of intervention, delegation, or coordination. Within the plan of services, the patient, significant other, agency, service organization, law enforcement agency, judicial system, or healthcare provider may be designated to implement interventions.

Plan of action. Comprehensive outline of steps to deliver services in order to attain expected outcomes and outputs.

Providers. Individuals, service organizations, agencies, and professionals with special expertise who provide services or assistance to patients.

Quality of care. The degree to which health services for patients, families, groups, communities, or populations increase the likelihood of desired outcomes and are consistent with current professional knowledge (ANA, 2004).

Scope of practice. An authoritative statement enunciated and promulgated by the profession that defines its practice, service, or education.

Significant other. Individual who is an intimate of and significant to the patient.

Standard. An authoritative statement, defined and promoted by the profession, by which the quality of practice, service, or education can be evaluated (ANA, 2004).

Standards of practice. Authoritative statements that describe a competent level of service in the profession, including assessment, diagnosis, outcomes identification, planning, implementation, and evaluation.

Standards of professional performance. Authoritative statements that describe a competent level of behavior in the profession, including quality of practice, professional practice evaluation, education, collegiality, collaboration, ethics, research, resource utilization, and leadership.

Summative evaluation. Those evaluative processes that result in an outcome or product (Weiss, 1998). Forensic nurses participate in continuous quality improvement utilizing the foundational processes identified in a summative evaluation.

Appendix B. Forensic Nursing: Scope and Standards of Practice (2009)

System. An assemblage of related elements that compose a unified whole, such as the legal and health systems, whose intersections provide the definitive context for forensic nursing, as well as the major systems in which forensic nurses practice:

- Healthcare (hospitals, surgery centers, community clinics)
- Investigative (medical examiner, law enforcement offices)
- Criminal Justice (district attorney, public defender offices),
- Correctional (jails, prisons, and detention centers)
- Government (military, local, state, provincial, and federal agencies)

Trauma. Injury which can be physical, psychological, emotional, spiritual, financial, or social; it can include loss of trust, safety, or security. Trauma is preventable and outcomes of trauma may be permanent or temporary. Trauma is amenable to independent or collaborative nursing intervention.

Victim. One who is acted upon and usually adversely affected by an outside incident. In forensic nursing, the victim may be the patient, the decedent, the perpetrator, the family, significant others, the suspect, the accused or falsely accused, the community, a population, a system, or the public in general.

REFERENCES

All URLs were retrieved April 13, 2009.

American Association of Colleges of Nursing (AACN). (1991). *Position statement: Physical violence against women.* Washington, DC: AACN.

American Association of Colleges of Nursing (AACN). (1998). *Essentials of baccalaureate education for professional nursing practice.* Washington, DC: AACN.

American Association of Colleges of Nursing (AACN). (2006). *The essentials of doctoral education for advanced nursing practice.* Washington, DC: AACN.

American Board of Nursing Specialties. (2005). *A position statement on the value of specialty nursing certification.* http://nursingcertification.org/pdf/value_certification.pdf.

American Board of Nursing Specialties. (n.d.). *Accreditation standards.* http://nursingcertification.org/pdf/ac_standards_short.pdf.

American Nurses Association (ANA). (2001). *Code of ethics for nurses with interpretive statements.* Silver Spring, MD: American Nurses Publishing.

American Nurses Association (ANA). (2003). *Nursing's social policy statement.* Washington, DC: Nursesbooks.org.

American Nurses Association (ANA). (2004). *Nursing: Scope and standards of practice.* Washington, DC: Nursesbooks.org.

American Nurses Association (ANA). (2005). *Recognition of a nursing specialty, approval of a specialty nursing scope of practice statement, and acknowledgment of specialty nursing standards of practice.* Paper presented at the Congress on Nursing Practice and Economics, Washington, DC.

Appendix B. Forensic Nursing: Scope and Standards of Practice (2009)

American Nurses Association (ANA) & International Association of Forensic Nurses (IAFN). (1997). *Forensic nursing scope and standards of practice.* Washington, DC: ANA.

Burgess, A. W., Berger, A. D., & Boersma, R. R. (2004). Forensic nursing: Investigating the career potential in this emerging graduate specialty. *American Journal of Nursing, 104*(3), 58–64.

Canadian Nurses Association (CNA). (2002). *Code of ethics for registered nurses.* http://www.cna-aiic.ca/cna/documents/pdf/publications/CodeofEthics2002_e.pdf.

Canadian Nurses Association (CNA). (2007). *Framework for the practice of registered nurses in Canada.* http://www.cna-aiic.ca/CNA/documents/pdf/publications/RN_Framework_Practice_2007_e.pdf.

Canadian Nurses Association (CNA). (2008). *Advanced nursing practice: A national framework.* Ottawa, ON: Canadian Nurses Association.

Canadian Nurses Association (CNA) & Canadian Federation of Nurses Unions (CFNU). (2006). *Joint position statement. Practice environments: Maximizing client, nurse, and system outcomes.* http://www.cna-aiic.ca/CNA/documents/pdf/publications/PS88-Practice-Environments-e.pdf.

Consensus Panel on Genetic/Genomic Nursing Competencies. (2006). *Essential nursing competencies and curricula guidelines for genetics and genomics.* Silver Spring, MD: American Nurses Association.

International Association of Forensic Nurses (IAFN). (2004). *Core competencies for advanced practice forensic nursing.* http://www.forensicnurse.org/associations/8556/files/APN%20Core%20Curriculum%20Document.pdf.

International Association of Forensic Nurses (IAFN). (2006). *IAFN vision of ethical practice.* http://www.iafn.org/displaycommon.cfm?an=1&subarticlenbr=56.

International Association of Forensic Nurses (IAFN). (2008). *History of forensic nursing.* http://www.forensicnurse.org/associations/8556/files/IAFN%20Presentation.ppt#283,4,history.

International Council of Nurses (ICN). (2004). *Position statement: Scope of nursing practice*. http://www.icn.ch/psscope.htm.

International Council of Nurses (ICN). (2006). *ICN code of ethics for nurses*. Geneva: International Council of Nurses.

Koop, C. Everett. (1986). *Public health and private ethics*. http://profiles.nlm.nih.gov/QQ/B/B/F/W/_/qqbbfw.pdf.

Ledray, L. E. (1999). *SANE development and operations guide*. http://www.ojp.usdoj.gov/ovc/publications/infores/sane/saneguide.pdf.

Lynch, V. A. (1990). *Clinical forensic nursing: A descriptive study in role development*. Unpublished thesis. Arlington, TX: University of Texas.

Mason, T., & Mercer, D. (1996). Forensic psychiatric nursing: Visions of social control. *Australian and New Zealand Journal of Mental Health Nursing, 5*, 153–162.

Merriam-Webster's collegiate dictionary, 11th ed. (2008). Springfield, MA: Merriam-Webster, Inc.

O'Carroll, P.W., & Public Health Informatics Competencies Working Group. (2002). *Informatics competencies for public health professionals*. Seattle: Northwest Center for Public Health Practice, University of Washington School of Public Health and Community Medicine.

QUAD Council. (2003). *Public Health Nursing Competencies* http://www.sphtc.org/phn_competencies_final_comb.pdf.

Schober, M., & Affara, F. A. (2006). *International Council of Nurses: Advanced nursing practice*. Malden, MA: Blackwell Publishing.

Sheridan, D. J. (2004). Legal and forensic nursing responses to family violence. In J. Humphreys & J. C. Campbell (Eds.), *Family violence and nursing practice* (pp. 385–406). Philadelphia: Lippincott, Williams & Wilkins.

Shives, L. R. (2008). *Basic concepts of psychiatric mental health nursing* (7th ed.). Philadelphia: Lippincott, Williams, and Wilkins.

Speck, P. M. (2000). *Things you didn't learn in nursing school: Forensic nursing principles - WHEEL.* Paper presented to the Emergency Nurses Association, Chicago.

Speck, P. M., & Peters, S. (1999). Forensic nursing: Where law and nursing intersect. *Advance for Nurse Practitioners, 11*(10).

National Nursing and Nursing Education Taskforce (N³ET). (2006). *A national specialisation framework for nursing and midwifery.* Melbourne, Australia: Health Workforce Australia. http://www.nhwt.gov.au/documents/N3ET/recsp_framework.pdf

United Nations. (1948). *Universal declaration of human rights, General Assembly resolution 217 A (III).* http://www.un.org/Overview/rights.html.

Weiss, C. H. (1998). *Evaluation* (2nd ed.), Upper Saddle River, NJ: Prentice Hall.

Index

Note: Entries flagged with [2009] indicate an entry from *Forensic Nursing: Scope and Standards of Practice* (2009), which is reproduced in this current edition as Appendix B. That information is not current; it is included for reference and historical context.

B

Baccalaureate degree, 25
Beliefs, practices, and communication
  patterns, 59
Benefits and costs. *See* Cost control
Body of knowledge in forensic nursing
  practice, 14, 24, 33

C

Canadian Nurses Association (CNA), 32
Care coordination, 33. *See also*
  Coordination of care
Caregivers, 47
  defined, 76
Caring
  defined, 76
Certificate programs, 28
Certification, 28, 30, 68
  defined, 76
Certified nurse midwives (CNMs), 27
Certified nurse practitioners (CNPs), 27
Certified registered nurse anesthetists
  (CRNAs), 27
Clinical decision support tools, 43
Clinical nurse specialists (CNS), 27
Code of ethics (nursing)
  defined, 76
*Code of Ethics for Nurses with
  Interpretive Statements*, 21–24;
  See also Ethics
  accountability and responsibility for
    practice (Provision 4), 23
  advocacy for the patient (Provision 3),
    22
  collaboration with the public and
    health professionals (Provision 8),
    23–24
  commitment to the patient
    (Provision 2), 22
  competencies involving, 57, 70
  duties to self and others (Provision 5),
    23
  nursing profession advancement
    (Provision 7), 23

nursing professional integrity
    and values and social justice
    (Provision 9), 24
  respect for the individual (Provision 1),
    22
  work settings and care and care
    environment contributions
    (Provision 6), 23
Collaboration, 6, 37, 62, 68. *See also*
  Communication
  competencies for, 62
  defined, 76
  Standard of Professional Performance,
    62
  (2009), 143, 192–193
Collaborative research and clinical
  inquiry, 67
Collegiality. *See also* Collaboration
  competencies for
  (2009), 142, 190–191
Commission for Forensic Nursing
  Certification, 26
Commitment to profession, 22
Communication, 6, 42, 61
  competencies for, 42, 44, 50, 51, 53,
    59, 61, 62, 64, 74
  skills, 61
  Standard of Professional Performance,
    61
Community
  defined, 76
Compassion, 22, 57
Competence
  cultural, 31
  defined, 76
  evaluation, 31
Competency(ies)
  assessment, 41–42
  (2009), 126, 182–183
  collaboration, 62
  (2009), 143
  collegiality
  (2009), 142, 190–191
  communication, 61
  consultation
  (2009), 134

assessment, 41, 43, 55
collection, 17, 19, 41, 42
defined, 77
dissemination, 42
evaluation data, 55
synthesis, 52
Data and information competencies, 41, 42, 43, 44, 49, 52, 57, 68, 69
Databases, 67
Death investigation
defined, 77
Death prevention, 37
Decision-making, 5, 23, 33, 50, 57, 59, 60, 63, 69
Delegation, competencies involving, 46, 63, 72
Desired outcomes, 62. *See also* Outcomes identification
Diagnosis, 5, 43–44
competencies for, 43–44
defined, 77
Standard of Practice, 43–44
(2009), 127, 183
Discrimination
based on gender identity, 24
based on sexual orientation, 24
Distance learning, 34
Documentation, 35, 36
competencies involving, 42, 43, 46, 48, 49, 51, 55, 62, 68
Domestic violence
defined, 77

E

Education, 3, 7, 10, 12, 15, 19, 25–26, 28, 29, 36
APRNs, 27
competencies for, 60, 62, 64–65
credentialing and, 26–27, 30, 32, 37
IAFN and, 16, 17, 28
international aspects, 32, 37
Standard of Professional Performance, 64–65
(2009), 140, 190
trends, 33–34
Educational preparation for forensic nursing, 28–29

Electronic medical records, 35
Empathy, 59
Environment
defined, 77
Environmental factors, 41
Environmental health, 7
competencies for, 74
defined, 77
Standard of Professional Performance, 74
Episodic care, 11
Ethical codes, 32
Ethical principles and priorities of forensic nurses, 24–25
Ethical work environment, 23
Ethics, 6, 11, 20, 21, 24–25; *See also* Code of Ethics for Nurses with Interpretive Statements, 25, 45, 57–58
competencies for, 42, 45, 50, 57–58, 63, 66, 67
and forensic nursing practice, 21–25
IAFN's *Vision of Ethical Practice*, 24, 57, 83. *See also Code of Ethics for Nurses with Interpretive Statements*
Standard of Professional Performance, 57–58
(2009), 144–145, 191–192
Evaluation, 6
competencies for, 45, 46, 54, 55, 60, 69
defined, 77
Standard of Practice, 55
(2009), 136–137, 186–187
Evaluation of competence, 30–31
Evidence-based assessment, 42
Evidence-based interventions, 49
Evidence-based practice, 31, 53, 60, 66
defined, 78. *See also* Evidence-based assessment; Evidence-based interventions; Evidence-based practice and research; Evidence-based strategies
Evidence-based practice and research, 10, 11, 19, 20, 21, 34, 26, 29, 30, 31, 37
competencies for, 42, 45, 47, 49, 50, 53, 60, 66–67, 69, 70, 72, 74

Institute of Medicine (IOM), 16, 33
Interdisciplinary colleagues, 67
International Association of Forensic
  Nurses (IAFN), 1–2, 4, 9, 10–11,
  16, 17, 24, 28, 31
  Vision of Ethical Practice, 24, 57, 83
International context of forensic nursing,
  32–33
International professional networks, 10
Interpersonal violence
  defined, 80
Interprofessional competencies, 20, 31,
  43, 48, 62, 68, 70
  defined, 80
Interprofessional education, 20, 34
Interprofessional healthcare, 44
  team, 52
Interprofessional teams, 42, 45, 47, 49,
  50, 51, 58, 60, 61, 63, 68
  defined, 80
Interventions, 1, 3, 11, 12, 27, 37
  culturally congruent practice and, 60
  implementation and, 49
  outcomes identification and, 45
  planning and, 47
  quality of practice and, 68
Intimate partner violence (IPV), 22
  defined, 80
  and forensic nursing, 15, 16–17
  *Intimate Partner Violence Education
  Guidelines*, 17

J

Joint Position Statement: Scopes of Practice,
  32

K

Knowledge
  defined, 80
Knowledge in forensic nursing, 2, 3,
  13, 14–15, 25, 26, 34, 36–37.
  See also Certification; Credentialing;
  Education
  APRNs, 27
  certification and, 76
  competencies involving, 41, 42, 59,
  63, 64, 66, 67, 68, 69

credentialing and, 26
education and, 28, 31, 64–65
forensic nursing roles and, 16, 17, 18
Knowledge, skills, abilities, and judgment,
  63, 66

L

Laws, statutes, and regulations, 35, 50,
  57, 72
Leadership, 6, 20, 31, 34
  competencies for, 48, 49, 50, 51, 52,
  60, 61, 62, 63, 68, 73
  role, 19
  Standard of Professional Performance,
  63
  (2009), 150–151
Legal
  defined, 80
  regulations, 35, 57, 72
Legal issues. *See* Laws, statutes, and
  regulations

M

Master's and doctoral education. *See also*
  Curricula/curriculum
  curricula for, 37
Measurement criteria [2009]
  assessment, 126, 182–183
  collaboration, 143, 192–193
  collegiality, 142, 190–191
  consultation, 134
  consultations, 134
  coordination of care, 132
  diagnosis, 127, 183
  education, 140, 190
  ethics, 144–145, 191–192
  evaluation, 136–137, 186–187
  health teaching and health promotion,
  133
  implementation, 131, 185–186
  leadership, 150–151
  outcomes identification, 128, 183–184
  performance appraisal, 189–190
  planning, 129–130, 184–185
  prescriptive authority and treatment,
  135
  professional practice evaluation, 141

Preventative death, 53. *See also* Death
Privacy, 62
Problem-solving tools, 42
Professional certification, 68
Professional commitment, 22, 25, 26, 29, 57, 58, 64
Professional competence in forensic nursing practice, 30–31
Professional practice evaluation, 7, 70–71
  competencies for, 70–71
  Standard of Professional Performance, 70–71
  (2009), 141
Professional trends and issues in forensic nursing, 33–37
  availability and access to forensic nursing services, 36–37
  forensic nursing education, 33–34
  forensic nursing research, 37
  global focus in forensic nursing, 37
  technological advances, 34–36
Psychiatric-mental health/correctional settings and forensic nursing, 18
Public health and forensic nursing, 19, 31, 37, 38, 57
  safety issues, 11, 13

Q

Quality
  care, 62
  defined, 81
  improvement, 68
  review processes, 23
Quality of care, 4, 20, 21, 23
  competencies for, 62, 63
  (2009), 188–189
Quality of life, 51
Quality of practice, 7
  competencies for, 56, 68–69
  Standard of Professional Performance, 68–69
  (2009), 138–139

R

Records and records storage, 35
Registered nurse (RN), 3, 25–27, 28
  defined, 82

Regulatory agencies, 30
Research
  collaborative, 67
  competencies for
    (2009), 146–147, 193–194
  skills, 67
Research-based practice, 66
Resource allocation, 72
Resource utilization, 7
  competencies for, 72–73
  Standard of Professional Performance, 72–73
  (2009), 148–149, 194–195
Respect, 57, 59, 62, 63
Risk management nurse, 19

S

Safety. *See* Patient, safety
SANE-A, 30
SANE-P, 30
Scope of nursing practice
  defined, 82
Self-care, 51, 58
Self-determination, 57
Self-evaluation, 25
Self-reflection, 58, 64
Sexual assault and forensic nursing, 15–16
Sexual assault nurse examiner (SANE), 16, 23–24
  defined, 82
Sexual Assault Nurse Examiner (SANE) Education Guidelines, 16
Sexual orientation, discrimination based on, 24
Social determinants of health, 41
Social justice, 24, 58
Socioeconomic status, 53
Specialty certification, 30
Spirituality, 53
Standards
  defined, 82
Standards of practice
  defined, 82
Standards of practice for forensic nurses, 39, 41–55
  assessment, 41–42
  coordination of care, 51–52